DASH DIET COOKBOOK FOR BEGINNERS

FOR BEGINNERS

Unlock Your Health Potential with 2000 DaysTasty Recipes & 28-Day Eating Plan to Lower Blood Pressure, Promote Weight Loss for Optimal Wellness.

Kellyann Brown

Table of Contents

THE DASH FOOD
PYRAMID

Introduction

This thorough introduction to the DASH diet is here to help you better your health and reach your ideal weight. The DASH diet can be exactly what you're looking for if you are looking to improve your nutritional intake and reduce your likelihood of cardiovascular disease. Dietary Approaches for Avoiding High Blood Pressure, or DASH, was created to help people in adopting a balanced diet and prevent hypertension. But the DASH diet can support healthy and permanent weight loss which has made it so well-liked. However, why has the diet known as DASH so successful? The answer arrives to give your body every component it requires to function efficiently. This book will teach you everything you need to know about the DASH diet, from its history and basics to how to follow it effectively. You are going to understand how the diet known as DASH could assist you achieve the weight you want and decrease your likelihood of cardiovascular disease, as well as helpful suggestions on how you can integrate it into your everyday life. Don't put off learning about how the DASH eating plan could assist you that achieving the good health and happiness that deserve!

WHAT IS THE DASH DIET?

The DASH approach to eating is an eating plan supports foods high in potassium, calcium, and magnesium, every one of which contributes to lower blood pressure levels. Additionally, a healthy lifestyle prioritizes whole foods rich in vital nutrients such as fiber, vitamins, and minerals, such as fruits, vegetables, whole grains, lean proteins, and low-fat dairy products. In contrast, the DASH eating plan limits sodium-rich meals like packaged meals, fast food, and processed food items. The dietary plan additionally limits the intake of saturated fats and cholesterol-rich foods like red meat, butter, and high-fat cheeses. It ought to be understood that the DASH diet does not require complete elimination of food categories and may be tailored to individual dietary preferences. If you like vegetarian food, for example, you can adhere to the DASH diet by eating plant-based proteins like beans, tofu, and nuts. Finally, the DASH diet was created after a long period of research by the National Heart, Lung, and Blood Institute (NHLBI) that demonstrated the efficiency of this nutritional plan.

Research conducted and published in the New England Journal of Medicine, in especially, discovered that the DASH diet can drastically lower blood pressure in just two weeks.

THE BENEFITS OF THE DASH DIET

Aside from reducing blood pressure, the DASH diet offers a number of other health benefits. For example, dietary changes can help lower the risk of heart disease, stroke, type 2 diabetes, cancer, and other chronic diseases. One of the reasons the DASH diet can reduce the risk of chronic diseases is that it is high in key micronutrients. For example, the DASH diet is abundant in fiber, antioxidants, minerals, and vitamins, all of which may safeguard the body from damage caused by free radicals and oxidative stress-related illnesses.

Additionally, the DASH diet could potentially minimize the risk of obesity. Because the diet prioritizes natural foods that are lower in saturated oils and added sweets, it can aid in calorie control and maintaining a healthy weight. The DASH diet may also be helpful for mental health. According to some studies, a nutritious diet such as the DASH diet can assist to reduce the probability of anxiety and depression. At last, the approach known as DASH can be customized to fit individual nutritional and lifestyle goals. The diet, for example, can be changed to meet the needs of people who are vegan or vegetarian and persons with intolerances to certain foods. Aside from decreasing hypertension, the DASH diet offers multiple health benefits. The DASH diet can help avoid a broad spectrum of long-term diseases, ranging regulate weight and enhancing mental health.

Lose weight in a healthy and sustainable way with the DASH diet

The DASH diet can help you lose weight in an effective and sustainable manner additionally decreasing the level of your blood pressure. Actually, the DASH diet was developed to assist people with implementing a nutritious lifestyle and managing hypertension. The DASH diet, with a focus on whole foods and nutrients, can help reduce the total amount of calories consumed while retaining satiety and taste. The DASH diet promotes a diet consisting of foods with fewer calories like vegetables, fruits, and grains that are whole while reducing the consumption of meals with many calories like deep-fried items and sweets. likewise, the DASH diet promotes sources of lean proteins, which include as white meat, seafood, legumes, and low-fat dairy products to help preserve satiety and lean body mass. Individuals in a study published in the Journal of the Academy of Nutrition and Dietetics who followed the DASH diet lost more weight than people who followed an ordinary low-calorie diet. In addition, DASH participants in the group showed a substantial decrease in fat in their abdomens, another form of body mass index associated with a situated probability of coronary artery disease and diabetes. A further advantage of the DASH diet is that it doesn't ask you to track calories or completely remove carbohydrates or lipids from your diet. However, it promotes the incorporation of foods that are nutritious whilst minimizing high-calorie and sodium-rich objects. Therefore, the DASH diet is a healthy and long-term choice for anybody who wants to lose weight while enhancing their health. In conclusion, the DASH diet can be a successful approach to losing pounds in a healthy and spanning manner. The DASH diet, with a focus on being filled with nutrients and low-calorie foods, can help reduce the total amount of calories consumed while preserving satisfaction and flavoring. likewise, the DASH diet is simple to follow and does not include the entire removal of every food group, which makes it a nutritious and environmentally friendly option for anybody looking to improve their health.

BLOOD PRESSURE

The DASH diet is a healthful solution for those at risk of cardiovascular diseases. How does it work? A nutrient-packed blend of fruits, vegetables, whole grains, low-fat dairy, fish, legumes, and nuts accomplishes the goal. Containing Vitamins C and E plus flavonoids and other essential nutrients beneficial to heart health, gastrointestinal tract, and even blood vessels – this diet packs a punch! Studies show that compared to standard diets the DASH could improve endothelial function by 19%. Wow! That's impressive. It helps regulate blood flow and keeps clots from forming – critical for maintaining good cardiovascular health. Did you know that the DASH diet has been linked to reducing inflammation and promoting heart health? It's no secret that blood pressure is a key factor for measuring cardiovascular health risks, but did you know what normal, prehypertension, hypertension, and malignant hypertension is classified as? Well, if you're under 18 years old then normal blood pressure is less than 120/80 mmHg. Prehypertension kicks in when your systolic blood pressure reads between 120-139 mmHg or diastolic measures between 80-89 mmHg. Upping the ante, we've got stage 1 hypertension at a systolic measure of 140-159 mmHg or diastolic reading at 90-99mmhg. Stage 2 hypertension takes it one step further reading perhaps 160/higher on the systolic scale or 100/higher on the diastolic side of things. But watch out; there's also malignant hypertension - a serious form of high BP associated with retinal hemorrhage and exudates.

Preventing hypertension

Hypertension, often known as hypertension of the arteries, is a serious - and all-too-common - condition.

High cholesterol can be a real heartbreaker, literally! It upping your risk of strokes and heart attacks, so it's essential to do whatever you can to curb it. Take those proactive steps now – trust me, you don't want something like this haunting your future. So what's the low-down? Several strategies can help keep hypertension at bay:

Wouldn't you know it - carrying extra pounds puts your blood pressure through the roof! Balancing the best in eating and getting regular exercise can help you keep your weight healthy, and lower your risk of hypertension. So don't give up, stay motivated and try to go for a walk every chance you get!

Woah - eating too much sodium can jack up your blood pressure. Cutting down on salt in your diet can help keep bp in check, though. You don't have to nix it - just try to limit the intake and you'll be good.

Let's get serious here: consuming a balanced diet rich in power foods - think juicy fruits, leafy greens, whole grains, lean proteins, and healthy fats - can help you stay fit and spruce up heart health. So don't hold back - incorporate these health benefits daily! Trust me; your body will thank you!

Wow, did you know that cutting back on booze can help keep your blood pressure in check? It's true - too much alcohol can ratchet up the pressure in your veins, so it's important to limit your drinking for good health.

Exercising regularly is a must if you wanna keep your weight in check and curb the risk of high blood pressure – no doubt about it! Just a few minutes of physical activity each day can make all the difference. So get moving and reap the rewards for years to come!

When we experience stress in our lives, it might momentarily boost our blood pressure. But don't worry; with the correct relaxation practices, such as meditation, yoga, and deep breathing, we can easily control our blood pressure! It only takes a quiet break from the daily hustle and bustle to maintain a healthy balance, so why not give it a try?

Managing your heart rate and blood pressure is essential, particularly if you are vulnerable to hypertension or have a family connection with it.

Your doctor may identify the possibility and give recommendations to help you avoid it.

BREAKFAST RECIPES
Apples Pancakes

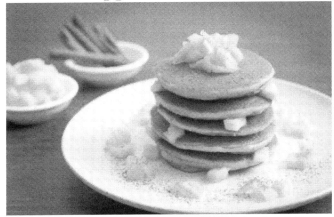

Preparation time: 10 minutes   **Cooking time:** 10 minutes   **Difficulty level:** Easy   **Servings:** 2

Ingredients:
- 1 apple
- 1 egg
- 1/2 cup of milk (about 120 ml)
- 3/4 cup of flour (about 80 grams)
- 1 teaspoon of baking powder
- 1 pinch of salt

Preparation:
Peel and dice the apple. In a bowl, mix the egg with the milk, flour, baking powder, and salt. Add the diced apple to the batter. Heat a lined skillet and pour in some batter. Fry the pancakes for 2-3 minutes on each side, until golden brown.

Nutritional values: Calories: 402 kcal   Protein: 14.1 g   Fat: 8.2 g   Carbohydrates: 70.8 g   Fiber: 5.1 g   Sugar: 22.7 g   Sodium: 382 mg

Porridge with banana and chocolate
Preparation time: 5 minutes Cooking time: 5 minutes **Difficulty:** Easy Servings: 1

Ingredients:
- 1/2 cup (40g) rolled oats
- 3/4 cup (200ml) milk
- 1 banana
- 1 teaspoon cocoa powder
- 1 teaspoon honey

Preparation:
In a pot, bring the milk to a boil and add the rolled oats. Cook on low heat for 3-4 minutes, stirring occasionally. Cut the banana into slices and add it to the porridge along with the cocoa powder and honey. Mix well and serve.

Nutritional values: Calories: 325 kcal Protein: 11 g Fat: 7 g Carbohydrates: 56 g Fiber: 7 g Sugar: 23 g Sodium: 80 mg

Walnut banana muffins

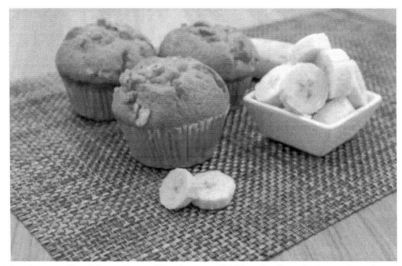

Preparation time: 10 minutes **Cooking time:** 25 minutes **Difficulty level:** Easy **Servings:** 6 medium-sized muffins

Ingredients:
- 2 ripe bananas
- 1 cup (100g) all-purpose flour
- 1/4 cup (50g) granulated sugar
- 1/4 cup (50g) unsalted butter, melted
- 2 eggs
- 1 teaspoon baking powder
- 1/2 cup (50g) chopped walnuts

Preparation:
Preheat the oven to 350°F (180°C).In a mixing bowl, mash the bananas with a fork. Add the flour, sugar, melted butter, eggs, baking powder, and chopped walnuts. Mix well until a smooth batter forms. Pour the batter into a muffin tin and bake for about 25 minutes, or until the muffins are golden brown. Remove from the oven and let cool before serving.

Nutrition facts (per muffin): Calories: 245 Fat: 13.5g Carbohydrates: 28.5g Protein: 5g Fiber: 2g

Fruit and vegetable smoothie

Preparation time: 10 minutes, **Servings:** 1, **Difficulty:** Easy

Ingredients:
- 1 banana
- 1 cup fresh spinach
- 1/2 cup fresh pineapple
- 1/2 cup fresh blueberries
- 1 cup skim milk
- 1 teaspoon honey
- 1/8 teaspoon salt

Preparation:
Place all the ingredients in a blender and blend until smooth and creamy.
Nutritional values per 1 smoothie: Calories: about 210 kcal Protein: 10 g Fat: 2 g Carbohydrates: 45 g Fiber: 7 g Sodium: 96 mg

Greek yogurt with fruit and granola

Preparation: 5 minutes, **Servings:** 1, **Difficulty:** Easy
Ingredients:
- 1/2 cup of low-fat Greek yogurt
- 1/2 cup of fresh fruit cubes (e.g. strawberries, blueberries, kiwi)
- 1/4 cup of unsweetened muesli

Preparation: In a bowl, mix the Greek yogurt with the fresh fruit cubes and unsweetened muesli.

Nutritional values for Greek Yogurt with Fruit and Muesli: Calories: around 200 kcal Fat: 2 g Carbohydrates: 33 g Protein: 16 g Fiber: 4 g Sugar: 17 g Sodium: 80 mg

It is a balanced and nutritious breakfast, rich in protein and fiber, which, thanks to the presence of fresh fruit, also provides a good intake of vitamins and minerals.

Whole wheat toast with peanut butter and banana
Preparation time: 5 minutes, **Servings:** 1, **Difficulty:** Easy

Ingredients:
- 1 slice of whole wheat bread,
- 1 tablespoon of natural peanut butter,
- 1/2 sliced banana

Preparation: Toast the whole wheat bread and spread the peanut butter on top. Add the sliced bananas on top.

Nutritional values for one serving of Peanut Butter and Banana Toast: Calories: 259 kcal Protein: 9 g Fat: 11 g Carbohydrates: 34 g Fiber: 6 g Sugar: 11 g Sodium: 208 mg

This recipe is a good source of complex carbohydrates, protein, and fiber, thanks to whole wheat bread and peanut butter, while the banana provides natural sugars and potassium. However, it icontrolling the amount of peanut butter used is important to its high-fat content.

Oatmeal and banana pancakes

Preparation time: 10 minutes, **Cooking time:** 10 minutes, **Servings:** 2, **Difficulty level:** Medium
Ingredients:

- 1 ripe banana
- 1/2 cup rolled oats
- 1/4 cup skim milk
- 1 egg
- 1 teaspoon baking powder
- 1/2 teaspoon ground cinnamon
- 1 pinch of salt
- 1/4 teaspoon of sodium

Preparation: Mash the banana in a bowl with a fork. Add the rolled oats, milk, egg, baking powder, cinnamon, salt, and sodium. Mix until a smooth batter forms. Heat a non-stick pan over medium heat. Pour the batter into the pan and fry the pancakes for about 2-3 minutes on each side until golden brown. Serve hot with maple syrup or fresh fruit.

Nutritional values for serving (without maple syrup or fresh fruit):
Calories: 229 Fat: 4 g Carbohydrates: 40 g Protein: 10 g m Fiber: 5 g Sodium: 171 mg

Vegetable frittata

Preparation: 10 minutes Servings: 2 **Difficulty:** easy
Ingredients:

- 4 eggs
- 1/4 cup skim milk
- 1/2 green bell pepper, diced
- 1/2 red bell pepper, diced
- 1/4 red onion, diced
- 1 cup fresh spinach
- 1/4 teaspoon salt
- 1/8 teaspoon pepper
- 1 teaspoon olive oil

Preparation: In a bowl, whisk the eggs with the milk, salt, and pepper. Add the peppers and onion and mix well. Heat the olive oil in a non-stick skillet over medium heat. Add the egg and vegetable mixture to the skillet and cook over medium heat for about 3-4 minutes, stirring occasionally. Add the fresh spinach on top of the frittata and cook for another 2-3 minutes, until the spinach is wilted and the frittata is cooked. Cut the frittata in half and serve hot.

Nutritional values per serving: Calories: 175 Protein: 14 g Fat: 11 g Carbohydrates: 6 g Fiber: 1 g Sodium: 340 mg

Scrambled eggs with avocado and tomatoes

Preparation time: 10 minutes **Servings**: 2 **Difficulty:** Easy
Ingredients:

- 4 eggs
- 1 ripe avocado
- 2 diced tomatoes
- 1/4 teaspoon of salt
- 1/8 teaspoon of pepper
- 1 teaspoon of olive oil

Preparation:

In a bowl, beat the eggs with salt and pepper, and heat the olive oil in a non-stick skillet over medium-low heat. Add the diced tomatoes and cook for 2-3 minutes until they become soft. Pour the beaten eggs into the skillet and gently stir with the tomatoes. Cook, stirring frequently, until the eggs are fully cooked. Cut the avocado into cubes and serve on top of the scrambled eggs.

Nutritional values per serving: Calories: 300 Protein: 16 g Carbohydrates: 12 g Fat: 22 g Sodium: 200 mg

Carrot walnut muffins

Preparation time: 15 minutes **Cooking time:** 20-25 minutes **Servings:** 6 Difficulty: Medium
Ingredients:

- 1 cup whole wheat flour
- 1/2 cup brown sugar
- 1 teaspoon ground cinnamon
- 1/2 teaspoon ground ginger
- 1/2 teaspoon ground nutmeg
- 1/2 teaspoon baking soda
- 1/4 teaspoon salt
- 1/4 cup sunflower seed oil
- 1 large egg
- 1 cup grated carrots
- 1/4 cup chopped walnuts

Preparation:

Preheat the oven to 180°C and line a muffin tin with paper liners. In a large bowl, mix together the flour, brown sugar, cinnamon, ginger, nutmeg, baking soda, and salt. In another bowl, beat the egg with the sunflower seed oil. Add the grated carrots to the egg mixture and mix well. Pour the egg and carrot mixture into the bowl with the dry ingredients and mix gently. Add the chopped walnuts and mix until well combined. Pour the batter into the muffin cups, filling them about 2/3 full, and bake for 20-25 minutes or until the muffins are golden and set in the center. Remove from the oven and let the muffins cool completely before serving.

Nutritional values per serving (1 muffin): Calories: 220 Fat: 11 g Sodium: 145 mg Carbohydrates: 28 g Fiber: 3 g Sugar: 13 g Protein: 4 g

Omelet with sweet potatoes and sausage

Preparation time: 15 minutes **Cooking time:** 30 minutes **Difficulty:** medium **Servings:** 4

Ingredients:

- 1 medium sweet potato, peeled and diced
- 1 tablespoon olive oil
- 1/2 medium yellow onion, finely chopped
- 2 turkey sausages, casings removed
- 8 large eggs
- 2 tablespoons skim milk
- 1/4 teaspoon salt
- 1/4 teaspoon black pepper
- 1/4 cup reduced-fat cheddar cheese, shredded

Preparation:

Preheat the oven to 400°F (200°C).Heat the olive oil in a non-stick skillet and cook the sweet potatoes and onion over medium heat until the potatoes are tender and the onions are translucent. Add the crumbled sausages and cook until no longer pink, about 5-7 minutes. In a medium bowl, whisk together the eggs, milk, salt, and black pepper. Pour the egg mixture into the skillet over the sweet potato and sausage mixture. Cook over medium heat until the eggs start to set around the edges, about 3-4 minutes. Sprinkle the cheese on top of the frittata and slide the skillet into the oven. Bake for about 10 minutes, or until the eggs are fully set and the cheese is melted. Remove from the oven and let the frittata rest for a few minutes before slicing into 4 portions and serving.

Nutrition values per serving (1/4 of the frittata): Calories: about 280 Protein: 18 g Fat: 16 g Sodium: 420 mg Carbohydrates: 22 g Fiber: 3 g

Chia seed pudding

Preparation Time: 5 minutes **Chilling Time:** 4 hours or overnight **Difficulty:** Easy **Servings:** 2

Ingredients:

- 1/4 cup chia seeds
- 1 cup unsweetened almond milk (or any milk of your choice)
- 1 tablespoon honey or maple syrup
- 1/2 teaspoon vanilla extract
- Fresh fruits, nuts, or granola for topping (optional)

Instructions:

1. In a bowl, combine the chia seeds, almond milk, honey or maple syrup, and vanilla extract. Stir well to ensure that the chia seeds are evenly distributed.
2. Let the mixture sit for about 5 minutes and then stir again to prevent clumping.
3. Cover the bowl and refrigerate for at least 4 hours or overnight. This will allow the chia seeds to absorb the liquid and form a pudding-like consistency.
4. Once the pudding has set, give it a good stir to break up any clumps.
5. Divide the chia seed pudding into serving bowls or glasses.
6. Top the pudding with your choice of fresh fruits, nuts, or granola for added flavor and texture.

Nutritional Information (per serving):

Calories: 180

Fat: 9g

Saturated Fat: 0.7g

Trans Fat: 0g

Cholesterol: 0mg

Sodium: 91mg

Carbohydrates: 20g

Fiber: 13g

Sugar: 5g

Protein: 6g

Pineapple smoothie

Preparation time: 5 minutes **Difficulty:** Easy **Servings:** 2

Ingredients:

- 2 cups fresh pineapple chunks
- 1 ripe banana
- 1 cup coconut milk
- 1/2 cup Greek yogurt
- 1 tablespoon honey or maple syrup (optional, for added sweetness)
- 1/2 cup ice cubes
- Fresh mint leaves, for garnish (optional)

Instructions:

1. Place the pineapple chunks, banana, coconut milk, Greek yogurt, honey or maple syrup (if desired), and ice cubes in a blender.
2. Blend on high speed until all the ingredients are well combined and you have a smooth and creamy texture.
3. Taste the smoothie and adjust the sweetness by adding more honey or maple syrup if desired.
4. Pour the smoothie into serving glasses.
5. Garnish with fresh mint leaves if desired.
6. Serve the Pineapple Smoothie immediately and enjoy its tropical flavors.

Nutritional values (per serving):

Calories: 210

Carbohydrates: 42g

Fat: 4g

Protein: 6g

Fiber: 4g

Sugar: 29g

Cinnamon cake

Preparation time: 15 minutes **Cooking time:** 40 minutes **Difficulty:** Easy **Servings:** 8-10

Ingredients:

- 2 cups all-purpose flour
- 1 cup granulated sugar
- 1 teaspoon baking powder
- 1/2 teaspoon baking soda
- 1/2 teaspoon salt
- 1 teaspoon ground cinnamon
- 1/2 cup unsalted butter, softened
- 2 large eggs
- 1 cup plain Greek yogurt
- 1 teaspoon vanilla extract

For the cinnamon sugar topping:

- 2 tablespoons granulated sugar
- 1 teaspoon ground cinnamon

For the glaze:

- 1 cup powdered sugar
- 2-3 tablespoons milk
- 1/2 teaspoon vanilla extract

Instructions:

1. Preheat the oven to 350°F (175°C). Grease and flour a 9-inch round cake pan.
2. In a mixing bowl, combine the flour, sugar, baking powder, baking soda, salt, and ground cinnamon.
3. Add the softened butter to the dry ingredients. Using an electric mixer or a stand mixer fitted with the paddle attachment, mix on low speed until the butter is well incorporated and the mixture resembles fine crumbs.
4. In a separate bowl, whisk together the eggs, Greek yogurt, and vanilla extract.
5. Pour the wet ingredients into the dry ingredient mixture. Beat on medium speed until the batter is smooth and well combined.
6. Pour the batter into the prepared cake pan and spread it evenly.
7. In a small bowl, mix together the granulated sugar and ground cinnamon for the topping. Sprinkle the cinnamon sugar mixture evenly over the cake batter.
8. Bake in the preheated oven for 35-40 minutes, or until a toothpick inserted into the center of the cake comes out clean.
9. Remove the cake from the oven and let it cool in the pan for 10 minutes. Then, transfer the cake to a wire rack to cool completely.

10. In a small bowl, whisk together the powdered sugar, milk, and vanilla extract to make the glaze. Adjust the consistency by adding more milk if needed.
11. Drizzle the glaze over the cooled cake.
12. Slice and serve the Cinnamon Breakfast Cake with a cup of coffee or tea for a delightful morning treat.

Nutritional values (per serving):

Calories: 330

Carbohydrates: 55g

Fat: 10g

Saturated Fat: 6g

Cholesterol: 65mg

Sodium: 290mg

Fiber: 1g

Sugar: 32g

Protein: 6g

French toast with fresh berries

Preparation time: 10 minutes **Cooking time:** 10 minutes **Difficulty:** Easy **Servings:** 4

Ingredients:

- 4 slices of bread (such as French bread or brioche)
- 2 large eggs
- 1/2 cup milk
- 1 tablespoon granulated sugar
- 1/2 teaspoon vanilla extract
- 1/4 teaspoon ground cinnamon (optional)
- Pinch of salt
- Butter or cooking spray, for greasing the pan
- Fresh berries (such as strawberries, blueberries, raspberries) for serving
- Maple syrup or honey for serving (optional)

Instructions:

1. Preheat a non-stick skillet or griddle over medium heat.
2. In a shallow bowl or pie plate, whisk together the eggs, milk, sugar, vanilla extract, ground cinnamon (if using), and salt until well combined.
3. Dip each slice of bread into the egg mixture, allowing it to soak for a few seconds on each side, making sure the bread is coated evenly.
4. Grease the preheated skillet or griddle with butter or cooking spray.
5. Place the soaked bread slices onto the skillet or griddle and cook for 2-3 minutes on each side, or until golden brown and cooked through.
6. Once the French toast slices are cooked, transfer them to serving plates.
7. Top the French toast with a generous serving of fresh berries.

Nutritional values:

- Calories: 250
- Carbohydrates: 35g
- Fat: 8g
- Saturated Fat: 3g
- Cholesterol: 120mg
- Sodium: 250mg
- Fiber: 3g
- Sugar: 10g
- Protein: 9g

Carrot and Almond Cake

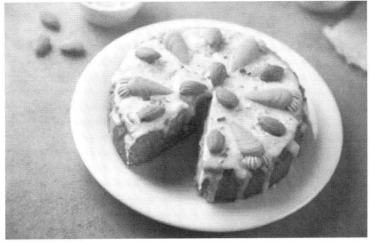

Preparation time: 20 minutes **Cooking time:** 40 minutes **Difficulty:** Moderate -**Servings:** 8

Ingredients:

- 1 1/2 cups grated carrots
- 1 cup all-purpose flour
- 1/2 cup almond flour
- 1/2 cup granulated sugar
- 1/4 cup brown sugar
- 1/2 cup vegetable oil
- 3 large eggs
- 1 teaspoon vanilla extract
- 1 teaspoon baking powder
- 1/2 teaspoon baking soda
- 1/2 teaspoon ground cinnamon
- 1/4 teaspoon ground nutmeg
- 1/4 teaspoon salt
- 1/2 cup chopped almonds, plus extra for topping
- Cream cheese frosting for serving (optional)

Instructions:

1. Preheat your oven to 350°F (175°C). Grease and flour a 9-inch round cake pan.
2. In a large mixing bowl, combine the all-purpose flour, almond flour, granulated sugar, brown sugar, baking powder, baking soda, ground cinnamon, ground nutmeg, and salt. Mix well.
3. In a separate bowl, whisk together the vegetable oil, eggs, and vanilla extract until well combined.
4. Gradually add the wet ingredients to the dry ingredients, stirring until just combined.
5. Fold in the grated carrots and chopped almonds, ensuring they are evenly distributed throughout the batter.
6. Pour the batter into the prepared cake pan and smooth the top with a spatula.
7. Sprinkle additional chopped almonds over the top of the batter.
8. Bake in the preheated oven for 35-40 minutes or until a toothpick inserted into the center comes out clean.
9. Remove the cake from the oven and let it cool in the pan for 10 minutes. Then transfer it to a wire rack to cool completely.
10. Once cooled, you can frost the cake with cream cheese frosting if desired, or serve it as is.

Nutritional values:

Calories: 320
Carbohydrates: 35g
Fat: 18g
Saturated Fat: 2g
Cholesterol: 55mg

Sodium: 220mg
Fiber: 3g
Sugar: 20g
Protein: 6g

Golden Oatmeal Waffles with Blueberry Compote

Preparation time: 15 minutes **Cooking time:** 20 minutes **Difficulty:** Moderate **Servings**: 4

Ingredients for the Waffles:

- 1 1/2 cups rolled oats
- 1 cup all-purpose flour
- 2 tablespoons granulated sugar
- 2 teaspoons baking powder
- 1/2 teaspoon baking soda
- 1/2 teaspoon ground cinnamon
- 1/4 teaspoon salt
- 1 1/2 cups buttermilk
- 2 large eggs
- 2 tablespoons melted butter (or coconut oil for a vegan option)
- 1 teaspoon vanilla extract

Ingredients for the Blueberry Compote:

- 2 cups fresh or frozen blueberries
- 2 tablespoons maple syrup
- 1 tablespoon lemon juice
- 1/2 teaspoon cornstarch (optional, for thickening)

Instructions:

1. Preheat your waffle iron according to its instructions.
2. In a blender or food processor, blend the rolled oats until they reach a fine flour-like consistency.
3. In a large mixing bowl, whisk together the oat flour, all-purpose flour, sugar, baking powder, baking soda, ground cinnamon, and salt.
4. In a separate bowl, whisk together the buttermilk, eggs, melted butter, and vanilla extract until well combined.
5. Pour the wet ingredients into the dry ingredients and stir until just combined. Do not overmix; the batter may be slightly lumpy.
6. Lightly grease the waffle iron with cooking spray or melted butter.
7. Pour the batter onto the preheated waffle iron, spreading it evenly, and close the lid.
8. Cook the waffles according to the instructions for your waffle iron until golden brown and crispy.
9. Meanwhile, prepare the blueberry compote. In a saucepan, combine the blueberries, maple syrup, and lemon juice. Cook over medium heat for about 5 minutes, stirring occasionally, until the blueberries soften and release their juices. If desired, whisk in the cornstarch to thicken the compote.
10. Remove the waffles from the iron and serve them warm, topped with the blueberry compote.

Nutritional values per serving (including the blueberry compote):

Calories: 380
Carbohydrates: 62g
Fat: 10g
Saturated Fat: 5g
Cholesterol: 107mg
Sodium: 527mg
Fiber: 5g
Sugar: 23g
Protein: 11g

LUNCH RECIPES
Zucchini Lasagna

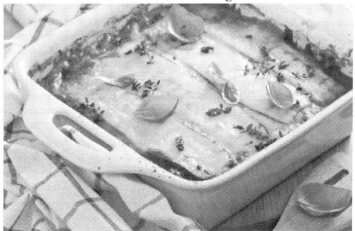

Cooking time: 1 hour **Preparation time**: 30 minutes **Servings**: 6 **Difficulty**: Medium **Special requirements**: Mandoline or sharp knife

Ingredients:

- 4 medium zucchini, sliced lengthwise into 1/4 inch thick strips
- 1 pound lean ground beef
- 1 medium onion, chopped
- 3 cloves garlic, minced
- 1 jar (24 ounces) low-sodium tomato sauce
- 2 tablespoons tomato paste
- 1 teaspoon dried basil
- 1 teaspoon dried oregano
- Salt and pepper, to taste
- 1 cup part-skim ricotta cheese
- 1/2 cup grated Parmesan cheese
- 1 egg
- 2 cups shredded part-skim mozzarella cheese
- Fresh basil leaves, for garnish (optional)

Instructions:

1. Preheat the oven to 375°F. Spray a 9x13 inch baking dish with cooking spray and set aside.
2. Using a mandoline or sharp knife, slice the zucchini lengthwise into 1/4 inch thick strips. Lay the zucchini strips on paper towels and sprinkle with salt. Let sit for 15 minutes to draw out excess moisture. Pat dry with paper towels.
3. In a large skillet, cook the ground beef over medium-high heat until browned. Add the onion and garlic and cook for 3-4 minutes or until softened.
4. Add the tomato sauce, tomato paste, dried basil, and dried oregano to the skillet. Season with salt and pepper to taste. Bring to a simmer and cook for 10-15 minutes.
5. In a small bowl, combine the ricotta cheese, Parmesan cheese, and egg. Season with salt and pepper to taste.
6. To assemble the lasagna, spread 1/4 of the meat sauce on the bottom of the prepared baking dish. Arrange a layer of zucchini slices over the sauce. Spread 1/3 of the ricotta mixture over the zucchini. Sprinkle with 1/3 of the shredded mozzarella cheese. Repeat the layers two more times, ending with a layer of meat sauce and mozzarella cheese.
7. Cover the baking dish with aluminum foil and bake for 45 minutes. Remove the foil and bake for an additional 10-15 minutes or until the cheese is melted and bubbly.
8. Let the lasagna cool for 5-10 minutes before slicing and serving. Garnish with fresh basil leaves, if desired.

Nutritional information per serving (1/6 of recipe):

- Calories: 320
- Total Fat: 15g
- Saturated Fat: 8g
- Cholesterol: 105mg
- Sodium: 660mg
- Total Carbohydrates: 13g
- Fiber: 3g
- Sugars: 8g
- Protein: 33g

Chicken and Vegetable Penne with Walnut Parsley Pesto

Cooking time: 25 minutes **Preparation time:** 15 minutes **Servings**: 4 **Difficulty**: Easy **Special requirements:** Food processor

Ingredients:

For the pesto:

- 1/2 cup chopped walnuts
- 1/2 cup chopped fresh parsley
- 1/4 cup grated Parmesan cheese
- 1 clove garlic, minced
- 1/2 teaspoon salt
- 1/4 teaspoon black pepper
- 1/4 cup olive oil

For the penne:

- 8 ounces whole wheat penne pasta
- 2 tablespoons olive oil
- 1 pound boneless, skinless chicken breasts, sliced into strips
- 1 red bell pepper, sliced
- 1 yellow bell pepper, sliced
- 1 medium zucchini, sliced
- Salt and pepper, to taste
- Lemon wedges, for serving

Instructions:

1. In a food processor, pulse together the walnuts, parsley, Parmesan cheese, garlic, salt, and black pepper until finely chopped. With the motor running, drizzle in the olive oil and process until smooth. Set aside.
2. Cook the penne according to package directions. Drain and set aside.
3. Meanwhile, heat the olive oil in a large skillet over medium-high heat. Add the chicken strips and cook for 5-6 minutes or until golden brown and cooked through.
4. Add the sliced red and yellow bell peppers and zucchini to the skillet. Season with salt and pepper to taste. Cook for 3-4 minutes or until the vegetables are crisp-tender.
5. Add the cooked penne to the skillet and toss to combine with the chicken and vegetables.
6. Divide the penne mixture among four plates. Drizzle each plate with the walnut parsley pesto. Serve with lemon wedges on the side.

Nutritional information per serving (1/4 of recipe):

- Calories: 530
- Total Fat: 26g
- Saturated Fat: 4g
- Cholesterol: 75mg
- Sodium: 510mg
- Total Carbohydrates: 44g
- Fiber: 8g
- Sugars: 5g
- Protein: 34g

Quinoa Salad with Chicken and Avocado:

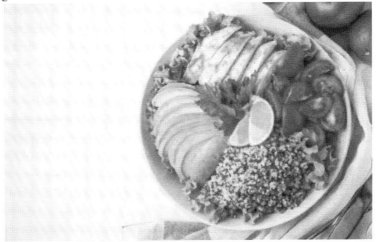

Preparation time: 15 minutes **Cooking time:** 20 minutes **Difficulty:** Easy **Servings:** 2

Ingredients:

- 1 cup cooked quinoa
- 4 oz grilled chicken breast, chopped
- 1/2 avocado, diced
- 1/4 cup red onion, chopped
- 1/4 cup fresh cilantro, chopped
- 2 tbsp lime juice
- 1 tbsp olive oil
- Salt and pepper, to taste

Preparation:

Cook quinoa according to package instructions and set aside to cool. Heat a grill or grill pan over medium-high heat. Season chicken with salt and pepper and grill until cooked through, about 5-6 minutes per side. Remove from heat and let cool before chopping. In a large bowl, combine the cooked quinoa, chopped chicken, diced avocado, chopped red onion, and chopped cilantro. In a small bowl, whisk together the lime juice, olive oil, salt, and pepper. Pour the dressing over the salad and toss to combine. Serve immediately or chill in the refrigerator until ready to serve.

Nutrition per serving (1/2 of recipe):

Calories: 349   Protein: 23 g   Fat: 18 g   Sodium: 134 mg   Carbohydrates: 27 g   Fiber: 8 g

Grilled Chicken and Vegetable Kabobs

Preparation time: 15 minutes **Cooking time:** 10 minutes **Difficulty:** Easy **Portions:** 4

Ingredients:

- 1 lb boneless, skinless chicken breasts
- 1 large zucchini, cut into chunks
- 1 red bell pepper, cut into chunks
- 1 red onion, cut into chunks
- 2 tbsp olive oil
- 1 tbsp dried oregano
- Salt and pepper to taste

Preparation: Preheat the grill to medium-high heat. Cut the chicken breasts into bite-sized pieces. Thread the chicken, zucchini, red bell pepper, and red onion onto skewers. Drizzle with olive oil and sprinkle with oregano, salt, and pepper. Grill for 10-12 minutes, turning occasionally, until the chicken is cooked through and the vegetables are tender. Serve hot.

Nutritional values per serving: Calories: 253   Protein: 28g Carbohydrates: 7g Fat: 13g Fiber: 2g Sodium: 94mg

Greek Salad with Grilled Shrimp Preparation

Cooking time: 10 minutes **Difficulty:** Easy **Portions:** 4

Ingredients:

- 1 lb large shrimp, peeled and deveined
- 1 tbsp olive oil
- 1 tbsp dried oregano
- Salt and pepper to taste
- 4 cups mixed greens
- 1 cucumber, chopped
- 1 pint cherry tomatoes, halved
- 1/2 red onion, thinly sliced
- 1/2 cup crumbled feta cheese
- 1/4 cup Kalamata olives
- 2 tbsp red wine vinegar
- 2 tbsp olive oil
- Salt and pepper to taste

Preparation:

Preheat the grill to medium-high heat. In a bowl, toss the shrimp with olive oil, oregano, salt, and pepper. Thread the shrimp onto skewers. Grill the shrimp for 2-3 minutes on each side, until pink and cooked through. In a large bowl, toss together the mixed greens, cucumber, cherry tomatoes, red onion, feta cheese, and Kalamata olives. In a small bowl, whisk together the red wine vinegar, olive oil, salt, and pepper. Drizzle the dressing over the salad and toss to combine. Divide the salad onto plates and top each with grilled shrimp. Serve immediately.

Nutritional values per serving: Calories: 240   Protein: 24g   Carbohydrates: 11g   Fat: 11g   Fiber: 3g
Sodium: 670mg

Turkey and Avocado Wrap

Preparation time: 10 minutes **Cooking time**: 0 minutes **Difficulty:** Easy **Portions:** 4

Ingredients:

- 4 whole wheat wraps
- 1/2 lb deli turkey, thinly sliced
- 2 avocados, sliced
- 1 red bell pepper, thinly sliced
- 1/4 red onion, thinly sliced
- 1/4 cup plain Greek yogurt
- 1 tbsp Dijon mustard
- Salt and pepper to taste

Preparation:

Lay the wraps flat on a clean surface. Divide the turkey, avocado, red bell pepper, and red onion among the wraps. In a small bowl, mix together the Greek yogurt and Dijon mustard. Drizzle the yogurt mixture over the ingredients in each wrap. Sprinkle with salt and pepper to taste. Roll up the wraps tightly and slice in half. Serve immediately or wrap in foil for later.

Nutritional values per serving: Calories: 363   Protein: 22g   Carbohydrates: 30g   Fat: 18g   Fiber:11g
Sodium: 625mg

Greek Salad with Chicken

Preparation time: 10 minutes **Cooking time:** 15 minutes **Difficulty:** Easy **Portions:** 4

Ingredients:

- 4 boneless, skinless chicken breasts
- 1 tbsp olive oil
- 1 tsp dried oregano
- Salt and pepper to taste
- 8 cups mixed greens
- 2 cucumbers, sliced
- 1 pint cherry tomatoes, halved
- 1 red onion, sliced
- 1/2 cup pitted Kalamata olives
- 1/2 cup crumbled feta cheese
- Juice of 1 lemon
- 2 tbsp red wine vinegar
- 1 tsp Dijon mustard
- 1 clove garlic, minced
- 1/2 cup extra-virgin olive oil

Instructions:

Preheat the oven to 375°F. In a baking dish, place the chicken breasts and drizzle with olive oil. Sprinkle the chicken with oregano, salt, and pepper. Bake for 15 minutes, until the chicken is cooked through. In a large bowl, combine the mixed greens, cucumbers, cherry tomatoes, red onion, olives, and feta cheese. In a small bowl, whisk together the lemon juice, red wine vinegar, Dijon mustard, garlic, salt, and pepper. Slowly whisk in the extra-virgin olive oil until the dressing is emulsified. Slice the chicken breasts and add them to the salad. Drizzle the dressing over the salad and toss to coat. Serve immediately.

Nutritional Information per serving: Calories: 459   Protein: 34g   Carbohydrates: 14g   Fat: 31g   Fiber: 4g Sodium: 807mg

Lemon and Garlic Chicken Pasta

Preparation time: 15 minutes **Cooking time:** 20 minutes **Difficulty:** Easy **Portions:** 4

Ingredients:

- 8 oz whole wheat spaghetti
- 1 lb boneless, skinless chicken breasts, cut into strips
- 1 lemon, zested and juiced
- 4 cloves garlic, minced
- 2 tbsp olive oil
- Salt and pepper to taste
- Fresh parsley, chopped

Instructions:

Cook the whole wheat spaghetti according to the package directions. Drain and set aside. Heat the olive oil in a large skillet over medium-high heat. Add the chicken strips and cook for 5-7 minutes, until browned. Add the minced garlic and cook for 1-2 minutes, until fragrant. Add the lemon juice and zest to the skillet and stir to coat the chicken. Add the cooked spaghetti to the skillet and toss to combine. Season with salt and pepper to taste. Serve hot, garnished with fresh parsley.

Nutritional values per serving: Calories: 330 Protein: 33g Carbohydrates: 27g Fat: 9g Fiber: 5g Sodium: 115mg

Chicken and Broccoli Alfredo Pasta

Preparation time: 15 minutes **Cooking time**: 20 minutes **Difficulty:** Easy **Portions:** 4

Ingredients:

- 8 oz whole wheat penne pasta
- 1 lb boneless, skinless chicken breasts, cut into strips
- 2 cups broccoli florets
- 2 cloves garlic, minced
- 1 cup low-fat milk
- 2 tbsp cornstarch
- 1/2 cup grated Parmesan cheese
- Salt and pepper to taste

Instructions:

Cook the whole wheat penne pasta according to the package directions. Drain and set aside. In a large skillet, cook the chicken strips over medium-high heat until browned. Add the broccoli florets and garlic to the skillet and cook until the vegetables are tender. In a small bowl, whisk together the milk and cornstarch until smooth. Add the milk mixture to the skillet with the chicken and broccoli and bring to a simmer. Cook for 2-3 minutes, until the sauce has thickened. Stir in the Parmesan cheese and season with salt and pepper to taste. Serve the chicken and broccoli Alfredo sauce over the cooked penne pasta.

Nutritional Information per serving:

Calories: 401 Protein: 39g Carbohydrates: 44g Fat: 10g Fiber: 7g Sodium: 341mg

Grilled Chicken and Vegetable Bowls

Preparation time: 15 minutes **Cooking time**: 20 minutes **Difficulty:** Easy **Portions**: 4

Ingredients:

- 1 lb boneless, skinless chicken breasts
- 1 red bell pepper, sliced
- 1 yellow bell pepper, sliced
- 1 zucchini, sliced
- 1 yellow squash, sliced
- 1 tbsp olive oil
- Salt and pepper to taste
- 2 cups cooked quinoa

Instructions:

Preheat a grill or grill pan to medium-high heat. Season the chicken breasts with salt and pepper and grill for 5-6 minutes per side, until cooked through. In a separate bowl, toss the sliced bell peppers, zucchini, and yellow squash with olive oil, salt, and pepper. Grill the vegetables for 3-4 minutes per side, until tender. To assemble the bowls, divide the cooked quinoa among four bowls. Slice the grilled chicken and add it to the bowls, along with the grilled vegetables. Serve hot.

Nutritional Information per serving: Calories: 342 Protein: 36g Carbohydrates: 29g Fat: 9g Fiber: 5g Sodium: 140mg

Lemon Garlic Shrimp Pasta

Preparation time: 10 minutes **Cooking time**: 20 minutes **Difficulty:** Easy **Portions:** 4

Ingredients:

- 8 oz whole wheat linguine
- 1 lb large shrimp, peeled and deveined
- 4 cloves garlic, minced
- 1 lemon, zested and juiced
- 2 tbsp olive oil
- Salt and pepper to taste
- Fresh parsley, chopped

Instructions:

Cook the whole wheat linguine according to the package directions. Drain and set aside. In a large skillet, heat the olive oil over medium-high heat. Add the shrimp to the skillet and cook for 2-3 minutes per side, until pink and cooked through. Add the minced garlic to the skillet and cook for 1-2 minutes, until fragrant. Add the lemon zest and juice to the skillet and stir to coat the shrimp. Add the cooked linguine to the skillet and toss to combine. Season with salt and pepper to taste. Serve hot, garnished with fresh parsley.

Nutritional Information per serving:

Calories: 299 Protein: 26g Carbohydrates: 29g Fat: 9g Fiber: 5g Sodium: 150mg

Turkey Meatball and Spaghetti Squash Bake

Preparation time: 20 minutes **Cooking time**: 50 minutes **Difficulty:** Medium **Portions:** 6

Ingredients:

- 1 large spaghetti squash, halved and seeded
- 1 lb ground turkey breast
- 1 egg
- 1/4 cup whole wheat breadcrumbs
- 1/4 cup grated Parmesan cheese
- 1 tsp dried oregano
- 1/2 tsp garlic powder
- 1/2 tsp onion powder
- Salt and pepper to taste
- 1 cup marinara sauce
- 1/2 cup shredded mozzarella cheese

Instructions:

Preheat the oven to 400°F. Place the spaghetti squash halves cut-side down on a baking sheet and roast in the oven for 30-35 minutes, until tender. In a large bowl, mix together the ground turkey, egg, breadcrumbs, Parmesan cheese, oregano, garlic powder, onion powder, salt, and pepper. Roll the mixture into meatballs, about 1-1/2 inches in diameter. Place the meatballs in a large baking dish and top with marinara sauce. Once the spaghetti squash is cooked, use a fork to scrape the flesh into spaghetti-like strands and add to the baking dish. Top with shredded mozzarella cheese. Bake in the oven for 20-25 minutes, until the cheese is melted and bubbly. Serve hot.

Nutritional Information per serving:

Calories: 213 Protein: 24g Carbohydrates: 11g Fat: 9g Fiber: 2g Sodium: 390mg

Lemon Herb Chicken and Whole Wheat Orzo Salad

Preparation time: 15 minutes **Cooking time:** 20 minutes **Difficulty:** Easy **Portions:** 4

Ingredients:

- 1 lb boneless, skinless chicken breasts
- 1 lemon, zested and juiced
- 2 cloves garlic, minced
- 1/4 cup chopped fresh parsley
- 2 tbsp chopped fresh basil
- 2 tbsp olive oil
- Salt and pepper to taste
- 8 oz whole wheat orzo
- 2 cups baby spinach
- 1/2 cup cherry tomatoes, halved

Instructions:

Preheat the oven to 400°F. In a small bowl, whisk together the lemon zest, lemon juice, garlic, parsley, basil, olive oil, salt, and pepper. Place the chicken breasts in a baking dish and pour the lemon herb mixture over the top. Bake in the oven for 20-25 minutes, until the chicken is cooked through. Meanwhile, cook the whole wheat orzo according to the package directions. Drain and set aside. In a large bowl, toss together the cooked orzo, baby spinach, and cherry tomatoes. Slice the cooked chicken and add it to the bowl with the orzo salad. Serve hot or cold.

Nutritional Information per serving:

Calories: 408

Protein: 36g

Carbohydrates: 39g

Fat: 11g

Fiber: 7g

Sodium: 172mg

Whole Wheat Penne with Grilled Chicken and Roasted Vegetables

Preparation time: 20 minutes Cooking time: 40 minutes Difficulty: Easy Portions: 4

Ingredients:

- 1 lb boneless, skinless chicken breasts
- 2 tbsp olive oil, divided
- Salt and pepper to taste
- 1 red bell pepper, seeded and sliced
- 1 yellow bell pepper, seeded and sliced
- 1 small zucchini, sliced
- 1 small red onion, sliced
- 2 cloves garlic, minced
- 1 tsp dried oregano
- 1/2 tsp dried thyme
- 8 oz whole wheat penne pasta
- 1/4 cup chopped fresh parsley
- 2 tbsp grated Parmesan cheese

Instructions:

Preheat the grill to medium-high heat. Brush the chicken breasts with 1 tablespoon of olive oil and season with salt and pepper. Grill the chicken for 6-7 minutes per side, until cooked through. Let rest for 5 minutes, then slice into strips. Preheat the oven to 400°F. In a large bowl, toss together the sliced red and yellow bell peppers, zucchini, red onion, garlic, dried oregano, dried thyme, and remaining tablespoon of olive oil. Spread the vegetables out in a single layer on a baking sheet and roast in the oven for 20-25 minutes, until tender and lightly browned. Meanwhile, cook the whole wheat penne according to the package directions. Drain and set aside. In a large bowl, toss together the cooked penne, sliced grilled chicken, and roasted vegetables. Top with chopped fresh parsley and grated Parmesan cheese.

Serve hot.

Nutritional Information per serving: Calories:434 Protein:36g Carbohydrates:45g Fat:12g Fiber:9g
Sodium:131mg

Mushroom and Chicken Risotto

Cooking time: 25-30 minutes **Preparation time:** 10 minutes **Servings:** 4 **Difficulty:** Medium Special requirements: Risotto pot

Ingredients:

- 1 tablespoon olive oil
- 1 finely chopped onion
- 2 cloves minced garlic
- 1 cup Arborio rice
- 1/2 cup white wine
- 4 cups vegetable broth
- 1 cup diced mixed mushrooms
- 2 chicken breasts, cubed
- 1/4 cup grated Parmesan cheese
- Salt and pepper to taste

Instructions:

1. Heat the olive oil in a risotto pot over medium-high heat. Add the chopped onion and minced garlic and cook for 2-3 minutes, or until the onion becomes translucent.
2. Add the rice and stir well to coat each grain of rice with the oil. Cook for 1-2 minutes, or until the rice becomes slightly golden.
3. Add the white wine and stir continuously until the wine has completely evaporated.
4. Gradually add the vegetable broth, one ladleful at a time, stirring constantly, until the risotto becomes creamy.
5. Add the mushrooms and chicken to the risotto and continue to cook until the rice is al dente and the chicken is fully cooked, about 5-7 minutes.
6. Add the grated Parmesan cheese and stir well.
7. Taste and adjust seasoning with salt and pepper as desired.
8. Serve hot.

Nutritional information per serving (1/4 of recipe):

Calories: 360
Total Fat: 9g
Saturated Fat: 2g
Cholesterol: 55mg
Sodium: 600mg
Total Carbohydrates: 44g
Fiber: 3g
Sugars: 2g
Protein: 24g

DINNER
Beef Stir-Fry with Broccoli and Brown Rice

Preparation time: 15 minutes **Cooking time:** 15 minutes **Difficulty:** Easy **Portions:** 4
Ingredients:

- 1 lb flank steak, thinly sliced
- 2 tbsp cornstarch
- 1/4 cup low-sodium soy sauce
- 2 tbsp hoisin sauce
- 1 tbsp honey
- 1 tbsp grated ginger
- 2 cloves garlic, minced
- 2 tbsp vegetable oil
- 1 lb
- 1 head broccoli, cut into florets
- 2 cups cooked brown rice

Instructions:

In a small bowl, whisk together the cornstarch, soy sauce, hoisin sauce, honey, ginger, and garlic. Add the sliced flank steak to the bowl and toss to coat. Heat the vegetable oil in a large skillet or wok over high heat. Add the marinated flank steak to the skillet and cook for 2-3 minutes, until browned. Add the broccoli florets to the skillet and stir-fry for an additional 3-4 minutes, until tender-crisp. Serve the beef stir-fry over cooked brown rice.

Nutritional Information per serving:

Calories: 407

Protein: 30g

Carbohydrates: 40g

Fat: 13g

Fiber: 5g

Sodium: 656mg

Mexican-Style Lamb Tacos with Avocado Salsa

Preparation Time: 20 minutes **Cooking Time**: 15 minutes **Difficulty:** Easy **Portions**: 4
Ingredients:

- 1 1/2 pounds ground lamb
- 2 teaspoons chili powder
- 1 teaspoon ground cumin
- 1/2 teaspoon smoked paprika
- 1/2 teaspoon garlic powder
- 1/2 teaspoon salt
- 1/4 teaspoon black pepper
- 8 small whole wheat tortillas
- 1 avocado, diced
- 1/2 cup chopped fresh cilantro
- 1/2 red onion, finely chopped
- 1 jalapeño pepper, seeded and finely chopped
- 1 lime, cut into wedges

Instructions:

1. In a large bowl, mix together the ground lamb, chili powder, cumin, smoked paprika, garlic powder, salt, and black pepper.
2. Heat a large skillet over medium-high heat. Add the lamb mixture and cook, stirring frequently, until browned and cooked through, about 10-12 minutes.
3. While the lamb is cooking, make the avocado salsa. In a small bowl, mix together the diced avocado, cilantro, red onion, jalapeño, and a squeeze of lime juice.
4. Warm the tortillas in the microwave or on a griddle.
5. To assemble the tacos, divide the lamb mixture among the tortillas and top with the avocado salsa. Serve with lime wedges on the side.

Nutritional Information per serving: Calories: 495 Fat: 28g Saturated Fat: 9g Cholesterol: 108mg Sodium: 605mg Carbohydrates: 29g Fiber: 8g Sugar: 3g Protein: 32g

Italian-Style Lamb Meatballs with Zucchini Noodles

Preparation Time: 30 minutes **Cooking Time**: 20 **minutes Difficulty:** Easy **Portions**: 4

Ingredients:

- 1 pound ground lamb
- 1/2 cup whole wheat breadcrumbs
- 1/4 cup chopped fresh parsley
- 1/4 cup chopped fresh basil
- 1/4 cup grated Parmesan cheese
- 1 egg, beaten
- 1 teaspoon dried oregano
- 1/2 teaspoon salt
- 1/4 teaspoon black pepper
- 2 tablespoons olive oil
- 4 medium zucchini, spiralized into noodles
- 2 cloves garlic, minced
- 1 can (14 ounces) diced tomatoes, undrained
- Salt and black pepper to taste

Instructions:

1. Preheat the oven to 400°F (200°C). Line a baking sheet with parchment paper.
2. In a large bowl, mix together the ground lamb, breadcrumbs, parsley, basil, Parmesan cheese, egg, oregano, salt, and black pepper until well combined.
3. Roll the lamb mixture into 20-24 meatballs and place them on the prepared baking sheet.
4. Bake the meatballs for 15-20 minutes, or until browned and cooked through.
5. While the meatballs are baking, heat the olive oil in a large skillet over medium heat. Add the spiralized zucchini and garlic and cook until the zucchini is tender, about 5-7 minutes.
6. Add the diced tomatoes to the skillet and simmer for 5-10 minutes, or until the sauce is heated through and slightly thickened.
7. Season the zucchini noodles with salt and black pepper to taste.
8. Serve the meatballs on top of the zucchini noodles with the tomato sauce spooned over the top.

Nutritional Information per serving: Calories: 505 Fat: 36g Saturated Fat: 12g Cholesterol: 151mg Sodium: 722mg Carbohydrates: 16g Fiber: 4g Sugar: 8g Protein: 31g

Grilled Chicken with Tomato and Cucumber Salad

Preparation time: 15 minutes **Cooking time:** 10 minutes **Difficulty**: Easy **Portions:** 4

Ingredients:

- 4 boneless, skinless chicken breasts
- 2 tbsp olive oil
- Salt and pepper to taste
- 2 cups cherry tomatoes, halved
- 1 English cucumber, diced
- 1/4 cup chopped red onion
- 1/4 cup chopped fresh parsley
- 2 tbsp red wine vinegar
- 1 tbsp olive oil
- 1 clove garlic, minced

Instructions:

1. Preheat the grill to medium-high heat.
2. Brush the chicken breasts with 2 tablespoons of olive oil and season with salt and pepper.
3. Grill the chicken for 4-5 minutes per side, until cooked through.
4. Meanwhile, in a large bowl, combine the cherry tomatoes, cucumber, red onion, and parsley.
5. In a small bowl, whisk together the red wine vinegar, olive oil, garlic, and salt and pepper to taste.
6. Pour the dressing over the tomato and cucumber mixture and toss to coat.
7. Serve the grilled chicken with the tomato and cucumber salad.

Nutritional Information per serving: Calories: 237 Protein: 29g Carbohydrates: 8g Fat: 10g Fiber: 2g Sodium: 91mg

Stuffed Bell Peppers with Ground Turkey and Brown Rice

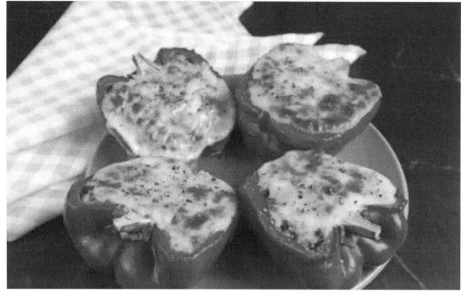

Preparation Time: 20 minutes **Cooking Time:** 50 minutes **Difficulty:** Intermediate **Servings:** 4

Ingredients:

- 4 bell peppers
- 1 lb. lean ground turkey
- 1 cup cooked brown rice
- 1 onion, chopped
- 2 garlic cloves, minced
- 1 can (14 oz.) low-sodium diced tomatoes
- 1 tbsp. dried basil
- Salt and pepper to taste

Instructions:

1. Preheat the oven to 375°F.
2. Cut the tops off the bell peppers and remove the seeds and membranes.
3. In a large skillet, cook the ground turkey over medium heat until browned.
4. Add the chopped onion and minced garlic to the skillet and cook for 2-3 minutes, until softened.
5. Add the cooked brown rice, diced tomatoes, dried basil, salt, and pepper to the skillet. Stir to combine.
6. Stuff the turkey and rice mixture into the bell peppers and place them in a baking dish.
7. Cover the baking dish with foil and bake for 30 minutes.
8. Remove the foil and bake for an additional 15-20 minutes, or until the bell peppers are tender and the filling is heated through.

Nutritional Information per serving:

Calories: 356

Protein: 27g

Carbohydrates: 32g

Fat: 14g

Fiber: 7g

Sodium: 305mg

Chicken Stir-Fry with Brown Rice

Preparation Time: 15 minutes **Cooking Time:** 20 minutes **Difficulty:** Easy **Servings:** 4

Ingredients:

- 1 lb. boneless, skinless chicken breast, cut into strips
- 2 tbsp. cornstarch
- 1 tbsp. vegetable oil
- 3 cups mixed vegetables (e.g. broccoli, bell peppers, carrots, snap peas)
- 1 tbsp. grated ginger
- 2 garlic cloves, minced
- 2 tbsp. low-sodium soy sauce
- 2 tbsp. honey
- 1/4 tsp. red pepper flakes
- 2 cups cooked brown rice

Instructions:

1. Toss the chicken strips in cornstarch until evenly coated.
2. Heat the vegetable oil in a large skillet or wok over medium-high heat.
3. Add the chicken strips and cook until browned and cooked through.
4. Remove the chicken from the skillet and set aside.
5. Add the mixed vegetables, grated ginger, and minced garlic to the skillet and stir-fry for 2-3 minutes, until the vegetables are crisp-tender.
6. Add the cooked chicken back to the skillet.
7. In a small bowl, whisk together the soy sauce, honey, and red pepper flakes. Pour the sauce over the chicken and vegetables and stir to coat.
8. Serve with brown rice.

Nutritional Information per serving: Calories: 392 Protein: 28g Carbohydrates: 56g Fat: 7g Fiber: 6g Sodium: 427mg

Quinoa and Black Bean Stuffed Bell Peppers

Cooking Time: 1 hour Preparation Time: 20 minutes Portions: 4 Difficulty: Easy

Special Requirements: Baking dish and foil

Ingredients:

- 4 bell peppers (any color)
- 1 cup quinoa
- 1 can black beans, drained and rinsed
- 1 small onion, diced
- 2 cloves garlic, minced
- 1 teaspoon chili powder
- 1/2 teaspoon cumin
- Salt and pepper to taste
- 1 cup low-sodium chicken or vegetable broth
- 1/2 cup shredded cheddar cheese (optional)

Instructions:

1. Preheat oven to 375°F.
2. Cut off the tops of the bell peppers and remove the seeds and membranes. Place the bell peppers in a baking dish.
3. Cook the quinoa according to package directions.
4. In a skillet over medium heat, sauté the onion and garlic until soft.
5. Add the black beans, chili powder, cumin, salt, and pepper to the skillet and stir to combine.
6. Add the cooked quinoa to the skillet and stir to combine.
7. Spoon the quinoa and black bean mixture into the bell peppers.
8. Pour the chicken or vegetable broth into the bottom of the baking dish.
9. Cover the baking dish with foil and bake for 45 minutes.
10. Remove the foil and sprinkle the shredded cheddar cheese on top of the stuffed bell peppers, if using.
11. Bake for an additional 10-15 minutes, or until the cheese is melted and bubbly.

Nutritional Information per serving (1 stuffed pepper):

Calories:255 Total Fat:4.5g Saturated Fat:1.5g Cholesterol:5mg Sodium:255mg Total Carbohydrates:44g Dietary Fiber:11g Sugars:6g Protein:13g

Roasted Vegetables with Goat Cheese Polenta

Cooking time: 40 minutes **Preparation time**: 20 minutes **Servings:** 4 **Difficulty:** Medium **Special requirements**: Large baking sheet, medium saucepan

Ingredients:

- 1 large eggplant, chopped into 1-inch pieces
- 1 large zucchini, chopped into 1-inch pieces
- 1 large red bell pepper, chopped into 1-inch pieces
- 1 large yellow onion, chopped into 1-inch pieces
- 2 cloves garlic, minced
- 2 tablespoons olive oil
- Salt and pepper to taste
- 1 cup yellow cornmeal
- 3 cups water
- 1/2 cup crumbled goat cheese
- 1/4 cup fresh parsley, finely chopped

Instructions:

1. Preheat the oven to 400°F.
2. Spread the chopped eggplant, zucchini, red bell pepper, and onion in a single layer on a large baking sheet. Drizzle with olive oil and sprinkle with minced garlic, salt, and pepper.
3. Roast the vegetables in the preheated oven for 20-25 minutes, or until they are tender and slightly caramelized.
4. In the meantime, bring 3 cups of water to a boil in a medium saucepan. Gradually whisk in the yellow cornmeal, stirring constantly to prevent lumps from forming.
5. Reduce the heat to medium-low and continue cooking the polenta, stirring frequently, for 10-15 minutes or until it has thickened to your desired consistency.
6. Remove the saucepan from the heat and stir in the crumbled goat cheese until it is fully melted and incorporated into the polenta.
7. Once the roasted vegetables are done, divide them evenly among four serving plates. Spoon the goat cheese polenta over the top of the roasted vegetables.
8. Sprinkle the chopped parsley over the top of the polenta.
9. Serve hot.

Nutritional information per serving (1/4 of recipe):

Calories: 305
Total Fat: 12g
Saturated Fat: 4g
Cholesterol: 13mg
Sodium: 145mg
Total Carbohydrates: 44g
Fiber: 8g
Sugars: 8g
Protein: 11g

Light Eggplant Parmesan

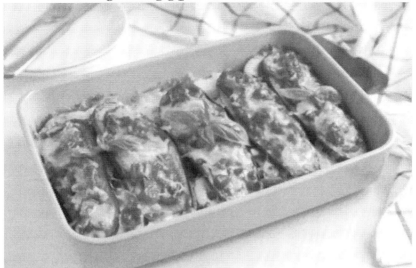

Cooking time: 50 minutes **Preparation time**: 30 minutes **Servings:** 4 **Difficulty:** Medium **Special requirements:** Large skillet, large baking dish

Ingredients:

- 2 medium eggplants, sliced into 1/4 inch rounds
- 1/4 cup all-purpose flour
- 2 eggs, beaten
- 1 cup whole wheat breadcrumbs
- 1/4 cup grated parmesan cheese
- 1 teaspoon dried oregano
- 1/2 teaspoon garlic powder
- 1/2 teaspoon salt
- 1/4 teaspoon black pepper
- 1 cup low-sodium tomato sauce
- 1/2 cup part-skim mozzarella cheese, shredded
- 2 tablespoons fresh basil leaves, chopped

Instructions:

1. Preheat the oven to 375°F.
2. In a shallow dish, whisk together the flour and a pinch of salt. In a separate shallow dish, beat the eggs. In a third shallow dish, combine the breadcrumbs, parmesan cheese, oregano, garlic powder, salt, and black pepper.
3. Dip each eggplant slice first in the flour mixture, then the egg mixture, and finally the breadcrumb mixture. Place the coated eggplant slices on a large plate.
4. Heat a large skillet over medium-high heat. Add enough oil to cover the bottom of the skillet. Once hot, add the coated eggplant slices in batches and cook for 2-3 minutes on each side or until golden brown. Place the cooked eggplant slices on a paper towel-lined plate to remove excess oil.
5. In a large baking dish, spread a thin layer of tomato sauce. Add a layer of eggplant slices on top of the tomato sauce. Spoon more tomato sauce over the eggplant slices and sprinkle with mozzarella cheese. Repeat the layering process until all the eggplant slices are used up. The top layer should be tomato sauce and mozzarella cheese.
6. Bake the eggplant parmesan in the preheated oven for 25-30 minutes or until the cheese is melted and bubbly.
7. Remove the eggplant parmesan from the oven and let it rest for 5 minutes before serving. Garnish with chopped fresh basil leaves.

Nutritional information per serving (1/4 of recipe):

Calories: 270
Total Fat: 9g
Saturated Fat: 3g
Cholesterol: 99mg
Sodium: 579mg

Total Carbohydrates: 34g
Fiber: 10g
Sugars: 10g
Protein: 17g

Mediterranean Quinoa Chicken Bowl

Cooking time: 25 minutes **Preparation time:** 15 minutes **Servings:** 4 **Difficulty:** Easy **Special requirements:** Large saucepan, medium skillet

Ingredients:

For the chicken marinade:

- 1 pound boneless, skinless chicken breasts, sliced into strips
- 2 tablespoons olive oil
- 1 tablespoon lemon juice
- 1 teaspoon dried oregano
- 1/2 teaspoon garlic powder
- 1/2 teaspoon salt
- 1/4 teaspoon black pepper

For the quinoa bowl

- 1 cup quinoa, rinsed and drained
- 2 cups low-sodium chicken broth
- 1 can (15 ounces) chickpeas, drained and rinsed
- 1 red bell pepper, diced
- 1/2 red onion, diced
- 1/2 cup kalamata olives, pitted and sliced
- 1/2 cup crumbled feta cheese
- 1/4 cup chopped fresh parsley
- Lemon wedges, for serving

Instructions:

1. In a medium bowl, whisk together the olive oil, lemon juice, oregano, garlic powder, salt, and black pepper. Add the chicken strips and toss to coat. Set aside to marinate while you prepare the quinoa.
2. In a large saucepan, bring the chicken broth to a boil. Add the quinoa, reduce the heat to low, and simmer for 15-20 minutes or until the quinoa is tender and the liquid has been absorbed.
3. Meanwhile, heat a medium skillet over medium-high heat. Add the chicken strips and cook for 5-6 minutes or until golden brown and cooked through.
4. In a large bowl, combine the cooked quinoa, chickpeas, diced red bell pepper, diced red onion, sliced kalamata olives, and crumbled feta cheese. Toss to combine.
5. Divide the quinoa mixture among four bowls. Top each bowl with the cooked chicken strips and chopped fresh parsley. Serve with lemon wedges on the side.

Nutritional information per serving (1/4 of recipe):

Calories: 540
Total Fat: 20g
Saturated Fat: 6g
Cholesterol: 80mg
Sodium: 920mg
Total Carbohydrates: 53g
Fiber: 10g
Sugars: 6g
Protein: 41g

Turkey Meatloaf

Preparation time: 15 minutes **Cooking time:** 60-65 minutes **Servings**: 6-8 **Difficulty level:** Easy

Ingredients:

- 500g ground turkey
- 1 egg
- 1/2 cup breadcrumbs
- 1/4 cup skim milk
- 1/2 chopped onion
- 1/2 cup chopped fresh spinach
- 1/4 cup chopped fresh parsley
- 1/4 cup grated Parmesan cheese
- Salt and freshly ground black pepper, to taste

For the glaze:

- 2 tablespoons ketchup
- 1 tablespoon apple cider vinegar
- 1 tablespoon honey
- 1 teaspoon Dijon mustard

Instructions:

1. Preheat the oven to 180°C. Line a baking dish with parchment paper.
2. In a large bowl, combine the ground turkey, egg, breadcrumbs, skim milk, chopped onion, chopped spinach, chopped fresh parsley, grated Parmesan cheese, salt, and freshly ground black pepper. Mix well with your hands to combine the ingredients.
3. Place the meat mixture into the prepared baking dish and shape it into a loaf.
4. In a small bowl, mix together the ketchup, apple cider vinegar, honey, and Dijon mustard. Spread the glaze on top of the meatloaf.
5. Cover the dish with foil and bake for 45 minutes.
6. Remove the foil and continue to bake the meatloaf for another 15-20 minutes, or until the internal temperature reaches 75°C.
7. Remove from the oven and let the meatloaf rest for 5-10 minutes before slicing and serving.

Nutritional values per serving (based on 6 servings):

Calories: 190
Fat: 6g
Carbohydrates: 14g
Protein: 21g
Fiber: 1g

SEAFOOD FIRST COURSES
Tuna and Tomato Linguine

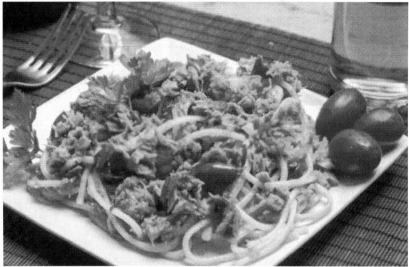

Preparation Time: 10 minutes **Cooking Time:** 20 minutes **Difficulty:** Easy **Portions:** 4

Ingredients:

- 12 oz whole-wheat linguine
- 2 tablespoons olive oil
- 1/2 onion, diced
- 2 cloves garlic, minced
- 1/2 teaspoon dried oregano
- 1/2 teaspoon dried basil
- 1/4 teaspoon red pepper flakes
- 1 can diced tomatoes (14.5 oz)
- 1 can tuna in water (5 oz)
- Salt and black pepper to taste
- 2 tablespoons chopped fresh parsley
- Lemon wedges for serving

Instructions:

1. Cook the linguine according to package instructions until al dente. Drain and set aside.
2. In a large skillet, heat the olive oil over medium heat. Add the diced onion and minced garlic, and sauté until the onion is translucent.
3. Add the dried oregano, dried basil, and red pepper flakes. Stir to combine.
4. Add the canned tomatoes (with their juice) to the skillet, and bring the mixture to a simmer. Cook for 10-15 minutes, or until the sauce has thickened.
5. Drain the can of tuna and add it to the skillet. Use a fork to break up the tuna into small pieces. Season the sauce with salt and black pepper to taste.
6. Add the cooked linguine to the skillet, and toss to coat with the sauce.
7. Divide the linguine among four plates, and sprinkle with chopped fresh parsley. Serve with lemon wedges on the side.

Nutritional Information per serving: Calories: 368 Fat: 10g Saturated Fat: 1g Cholesterol: 7mg Sodium: 319mg Carbohydrates: 52g Fiber: 10g Sugar: 7g Protein: 20g

Fish and Spinach Lasagna

Preparation time: 30 minutes **Cooking time:** 45 minutes **Difficulty:** Moderate Portions: 8

Ingredients:

- 12 whole-wheat lasagna noodles
- 1 tbsp olive oil
- 1 large onion, chopped
- 3 cloves garlic, minced
- 2 cans (14.5 oz) diced tomatoes, undrained
- 2 tbsp tomato paste
- 1/4 cup chopped fresh basil
- 1/4 tsp red pepper flakes
- 1 lb fresh spinach, chopped
- 1 lb white fish, such as cod or halibut, cut into bite-sized pieces
- 2 cups part-skim ricotta cheese
- 1/4 cup grated Parmesan cheese
- 1 egg
- Salt and pepper to taste
- Cooking spray

Instructions:

1. Preheat the oven to 375°F (190°C).
2. Cook the lasagna noodles according to package directions. Drain and set aside.
3. In a large skillet, heat the olive oil over medium heat. Add the onion and garlic and cook for 3-4 minutes, or until softened.
4. Add the diced tomatoes, tomato paste, basil, and red pepper flakes to the skillet. Stir to combine and simmer for 10 minutes.
5. Add the chopped spinach and fish to the skillet. Stir gently to coat with the tomato sauce and cook for 2-3 minutes, or until the fish is cooked through.
6. In a medium bowl, combine the ricotta cheese, Parmesan cheese, egg, salt, and pepper.
7. Spray a 9x13 inch baking dish with cooking spray. Spread 1/4 cup of the tomato sauce on the bottom of the dish.
8. Arrange 4 lasagna noodles over the tomato sauce in the dish. Top with 1/3 of the fish and spinach mixture.
9. Spoon 1/3 of the ricotta cheese mixture over the fish and spinach mixture.
10. Repeat layers twice more, ending with a layer of lasagna noodles.
11. Spoon the remaining tomato sauce over the top of the lasagna.
12. Cover the dish with foil and bake for 30 minutes.
13. Remove the foil and bake for an additional 10-15 minutes, or until the cheese is melted and bubbly.
14. Let the lasagna cool for 10-15 minutes before serving.

Nutrition information per serving:

Calories: 390

Fat: 12g

Saturated Fat: 5g

Cholesterol: 85mg

Sodium: 520mg

Carbohydrates:35g

 Fiber: 6g

Sugar: 9g

Protein:34g

Orange risotto with swordfish and shrimp

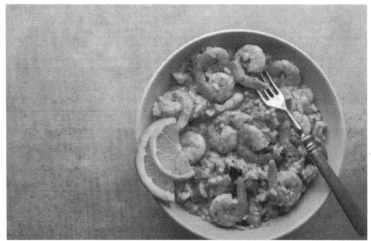

Preparation time: 10 minutes **Cooking time:** 40 minutes **Difficulty:** Moderate **Portions:** 4

Ingredients:

- 1 lb swordfish, cut into bite-sized pieces
- 1 lb shrimp, peeled and deveined
- 1 tbsp olive oil
- 1 onion, chopped
- 2 cloves garlic, minced
- 2 cups Arborio rice
- 1/2 cup dry white wine
- 5 cups low-sodium chicken or vegetable broth
- Juice and zest of 2 oranges
- 1/2 cup grated Parmesan cheese
- Salt and pepper to taste
- Chopped parsley for garnish

Instructions:

1. In a large skillet, heat the olive oil over medium heat. Add the onion and garlic and cook for 3-4 minutes, or until softened.
2. Add the swordfish and shrimp to the skillet. Cook for 2-3 minutes, or until the seafood is cooked through. Remove from the skillet and set aside.
3. In the same skillet, add the Arborio rice and stir to coat with the remaining oil. Cook for 1-2 minutes, or until the rice is lightly toasted.
4. Add the white wine to the skillet and stir until absorbed.
5. Add the chicken or vegetable broth, 1/2 cup at a time, stirring constantly until each addition is absorbed before adding more. Continue this process for 20-25 minutes, or until the rice is tender and the mixture is creamy.
6. Stir in the orange juice and zest, Parmesan cheese, and salt and pepper to taste.
7. Add the cooked swordfish and shrimp to the skillet and stir to combine.
8. Serve the risotto hot, garnished with chopped parsley.

Nutrition information per serving: Calories:500 Fat:10g Saturated Fat:3g Cholesterol:200mg
Sodium:520mg Carbohydrates:63g Fiber:3g Sugar:5g Protein:36g

Spaghetti with fish balls

Preparation time: 20 minutes **Cooking time**: 30 minutes **Difficulty:** Moderate **Portions**: 4

Ingredients:

- 1 lb spaghetti
- 1 lb white fish fillets (such as cod or haddock)
- 1 onion, chopped
- 2 cloves garlic, minced
- 1 egg, lightly beaten
- 1/2 cup breadcrumbs
- 1/4 cup chopped fresh parsley
- 1/4 tsp dried oregano
- Salt and pepper to taste
- 2 tbsp olive oil
- 1 can (14.5 oz) diced tomatoes
- 1/2 cup low-sodium chicken or vegetable broth
- 1/4 cup chopped fresh basil

Instructions:

1. Cook the spaghetti according to the package directions. Drain and set aside.
2. In a food processor, pulse the fish fillets until finely chopped.
3. In a bowl, mix together the chopped fish, onion, garlic, egg, breadcrumbs, parsley, oregano, salt, and pepper.
4. Form the mixture into 1-inch balls.
5. Heat the olive oil in a large skillet over medium heat. Add the fish balls and cook for 5-6 minutes, or until browned on all sides.
6. Add the diced tomatoes and chicken or vegetable broth to the skillet. Bring to a simmer and cook for 15-20 minutes, or until the sauce has thickened slightly and the fish balls are cooked through.
7. Serve the spaghetti topped with the fish balls and sauce, garnished with chopped fresh basil.

Nutrition information per serving:

Calories: 490
Fat: 10g
Saturated Fat: 2g
Cholesterol: 130mg
Sodium: 320mg
Carbohydrates: 67g
Fiber: 5g
Sugar: 5g
Protein: 34g

Venus rice with shrimps and zucchini

Preparation time: 10 minutes **Cooking time:** 25 minutes **Difficulty:** Easy **Portions:** 4

Ingredients:

- 1 cup Venus rice (or any whole grain rice)
- 1 3/4 cups low-sodium chicken or vegetable broth
- 1 tbsp olive oil
- 1 onion, chopped
- 2 cloves garlic, minced
- 2 zucchinis, diced
- 1/2 lb shrimp, peeled and deveined
- 1/4 tsp dried thyme
- Salt and pepper to taste
- 1/4 cup chopped fresh parsley
- Lemon wedges for serving

Instructions:

1. Rinse the Venus rice in cold water and drain.
2. In a medium saucepan, combine the Venus rice and chicken or vegetable broth. Bring to a boil, then reduce heat to low, cover, and simmer for 20-25 minutes, or until the rice is tender and the liquid is absorbed.
3. Meanwhile, in a large skillet, heat the olive oil over medium heat. Add the onion and garlic and cook for 2-3 minutes, or until softened.
4. Add the diced zucchinis and cook for 3-4 minutes, or until softened.
5. Add the shrimp and thyme to the skillet. Cook for 3-4 minutes, or until the shrimp are pink and cooked through.
6. Season with salt and pepper to taste. Stir in the chopped parsley.
7. Serve the Venus rice topped with the shrimp and zucchini mixture, with lemon wedges on the side.

Nutrition information per serving: Calories:310   Fat:6g   Saturated Fat:1g   Cholesterol:95mg   Sodium:190mg   Carbohydrates:46g   Fiber:3g   Sugar:4g   Protein:18g

Fish couscous

This fish couscous recipe is a great source of lean protein, fiber, and healthy carbohydrates. It's also low in saturated fat and sodium.

Preparation time: 15 minutes **Cooking time:** 30 minutes **Difficulty:** Easy **Portions:** 4

Ingredients:

- 1 lb fish fillets (such as cod or tilapia), cut into bite-sized pieces
- 1 onion, chopped
- 2 cloves garlic, minced
- 1 red bell pepper, chopped
- 1 yellow bell pepper, chopped
- 1 zucchini, chopped
- 1 can (14 oz) diced tomatoes
- 1 tbsp tomato paste
- 1 tsp ground cumin
- 1 tsp ground coriander
- 1/2 tsp paprika
- 1/4 tsp cayenne pepper (optional)
- 1/2 cup low-sodium chicken or vegetable broth
- 1 cup whole wheat couscous
- Salt and pepper to taste
- Lemon wedges for serving

Instructions:

1. In a large skillet, heat 1 tablespoon of olive oil over medium heat. Add the onion and garlic and cook for 2-3 minutes, or until softened.
2. Add the red and yellow bell peppers and zucchini. Cook for 5-7 minutes, or until softened.
3. Add the diced tomatoes, tomato paste, cumin, coriander, paprika, and cayenne pepper (if using). Stir to combine.
4. Add the fish pieces to the skillet, stirring gently to coat with the tomato and vegetable mixture.
5. Pour the chicken or vegetable broth over the fish mixture. Cover and simmer for 10-15 minutes, or until the fish is cooked through.
6. Meanwhile, prepare the couscous according to package instructions.

7. Fluff the couscous with a fork and divide it among four plates.
8. Spoon the fish and vegetable mixture over the couscous.
9. Serve with lemon wedges on the side.

Nutritional information (per serving):

Calories: 325 kcal

Fat: 6.5 g

Saturated Fat: 1 g

Cholesterol: 65 mg

Sodium: 275 mg

Carbohydrates: 39 g

Fiber: 7 g

Sugar: 7 g

Protein: 29 g

Pad Thai with shrimp

Preparation time: 20 minutes **Cooking time**: 15 minutes **Difficulty**: Easy **Portions**: 4

Ingredients:
- 8 oz rice noodles
- 1 lb medium shrimp, peeled and deveined
- 3 cloves garlic, minced
- 2 shallots, finely sliced
- 1/4 cup low-sodium chicken or vegetable broth
- 2 tbsp low-sodium soy sauce
- 2 tbsp lime juice
- 1 tbsp brown sugar
- 2 tbsp vegetable oil
- 2 eggs, lightly beaten
- 2 cups bean sprouts
- 2 green onions, sliced
- 1/4 cup chopped roasted unsalted peanuts
- 2 tbsp chopped fresh cilantro

Instructions:
1. Cook the rice noodles according to package instructions. Drain and set aside.
2. In a small bowl, whisk together the chicken or vegetable broth, soy sauce, lime juice, and brown sugar. Set aside.
3. In a wok or large skillet, heat the vegetable oil over medium-high heat. Add the garlic and shallots and cook for 1-2 minutes, or until fragrant.
4. Add the shrimp and cook for 2-3 minutes, or until pink and cooked through.
5. Push the shrimp to one side of the wok or skillet and add the beaten eggs to the other side. Scramble the eggs until just cooked, then mix in with the shrimp.
6. Add the cooked rice noodles to the wok or skillet and pour the sauce over everything. Toss everything together until the noodles are coated with the sauce.
7. Add the bean sprouts and green onions, and stir to combine.
8. Divide the Pad Thai among four plates and top with chopped peanuts and cilantro.

Nutritional information (per serving):
- Calories: 420 kcal
- Fat: 14 g
- Saturated Fat: 2 g
- Cholesterol: 275 mg
- Sodium: 610 mg
- Carbohydrates: 48 g
- Fiber: 3 g
- Sugar: 8 g
- Protein: 26 g

SEAFOOD MAIN COURSES

Warm Potato and Octopus Salad with Sweet Potatoes

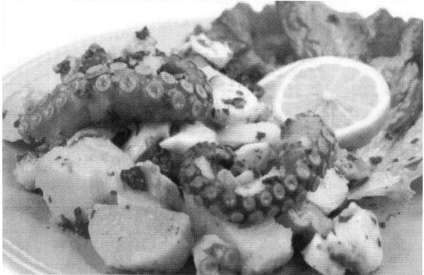

Cooking time: 40 minutes **Preparation time**: 20 minutes **Servings**: 4 Difficulty: **Medium Special requirements**: Large pot, oven-safe skillet or baking dish

Ingredients:

- 1 lb octopus
- 2 large potatoes, peeled and chopped into small cubes
- 2 large sweet potatoes, peeled and chopped into small cubes
- 2 tablespoons olive oil
- 1/2 red onion, thinly sliced
- 1/4 cup fresh parsley, finely chopped
- Salt and pepper to taste

Instructions:

1. Preheat the oven to 375°F.
2. Bring a large pot of salted water to a boil. Add the octopus and boil for 20-25 minutes, or until the octopus is tender. Drain and rinse the octopus, then chop it into bite-sized pieces.
3. In the meantime, in a separate pot, cook the chopped potatoes and sweet potatoes in salted water for 10-12 minutes or until they are tender but still hold their shape. Drain and set aside.
4. Heat the olive oil in an oven-safe skillet or baking dish over medium-high heat. Add the sliced red onion and cook for 3-4 minutes, or until the onion is soft and translucent.
5. Add the chopped octopus to the skillet and cook for an additional 3-4 minutes, or until the octopus is slightly browned.
6. Add the cooked potatoes and sweet potatoes to the skillet and stir well to combine with the octopus and onion.
7. Place the skillet in the preheated oven and bake for 10-12 minutes, or until the potatoes are slightly crispy.
8. Remove the skillet from the oven and sprinkle the chopped parsley over the top of the salad.
9. Serve warm.

Nutritional information per serving (1/4 of recipe):

Calories: 285
Total Fat: 7g
Saturated Fat: 1g
Cholesterol: 35mg
Sodium: 260mg

Total Carbohydrates: 38g
Fiber: 6g
Sugars: 8g
Protein: 17g

Grilled Salmon with Mango Salsa

Cooking Time: 15 minutes **Preparation Time:** 20 minutes **Portions:** 4 **Difficulty:** Easy
Special Requirements: Grill or grill pan

Ingredients:

- 4 salmon fillets (4-6 ounces each)
- 1 ripe mango, peeled and diced
- 1 small red onion, diced
- 1/4 cup chopped fresh cilantro
- 1 jalapeño pepper, seeded and minced
- 1 lime, juiced
- Salt and pepper to taste

Instructions:

1. Preheat grill or grill pan to medium-high heat.
2. Season the salmon fillets with salt and pepper.
3. Grill the salmon fillets for 3-4 minutes per side, or until cooked through
4. In a bowl, combine the diced mango, red onion, cilantro, jalapeño pepper, lime juice, salt, and pepper.
5. Serve the grilled salmon with the mango salsa on top.

Nutritional Information per serving (1 salmon fillet with salsa):

Calories: 265
Total Fat: 12g
Saturated Fat: 2g
Cholesterol: 80mg
Sodium: 100mg
Total Carbohydrates: 10g
Dietary Fiber: 2g
Sugars: 7g
Protein: 29g

Tuna meatloaf

Preparation time: 10 minutes **Cooking time:** 30-35 minutes **Servings:** 4-6 **Difficulty level:** Easy

Ingredients:

- 2 cans (12 oz each) of tuna in water, drained
- 1/2 cup of whole wheat breadcrumbs
- 1/4 cup of nonfat milk
- 1/4 cup of finely chopped red onion
- 1/4 cup of chopped parsley
- 2 tablespoons of lemon juice
- 1 egg
- Salt and freshly ground black pepper, to taste

For the glaze:
- 2 tablespoons of ketchup
- 1 tablespoon of apple cider vinegar
- 1 tablespoon of honey
- 1 teaspoon of Dijon mustard

Preparation:

1. Preheat oven to 375°F. Lightly grease a loaf pan with cooking spray.
2. In a large bowl, combine tuna, breadcrumbs, milk, red onion, parsley, lemon juice, egg, salt and pepper. Mix well with your hands.
3. Press the mixture into the loaf pan, making sure to pack it down tightly.
4. In a small bowl, whisk together ketchup, apple cider vinegar, honey, and Dijon mustard. Spread the glaze over the top of the tuna mixture.
5. Bake for 30-35 minutes, or until the loaf is cooked through and the glaze is golden brown.
6. Let the tuna loaf cool in the pan for 5-10 minutes, then transfer to a cutting board and slice into servings.

Nutritional values (per serving):

Calories: 180
Fat 2g
Carbohydrates: 12g

Protein: 29g
Fiber: 2g

Almond-Crusted Cod with Asparagus

Preparation time: 10 minutes **Cooking time:** 25 minutes **Servings:** 4 **Difficulty:** Easy

Ingredients:

- 4 cod fillets (about 6 oz. each)
- 1/2 cup almond flour
- 1/2 cup sliced almonds
- 2 cloves garlic, minced
- 2 tablespoons chopped parsley
- Salt and pepper
- 1 egg, beaten
- 1 bunch asparagus, trimmed
- 1 tablespoon olive oil

Preparation:

1. Preheat the oven to 375°F (190°C).
2. Season the cod fillets with salt and pepper.
3. In a bowl, mix together the almond flour, sliced almonds, minced garlic, chopped parsley, and a pinch of salt and pepper.
4. Dip each cod fillet in the beaten egg and then coat it with the almond mixture, pressing it onto the fillet to adhere.
5. Place the coated fillets onto a baking sheet lined with parchment paper.
6. Bake for 15-20 minutes, until the crust is golden brown and the fish is cooked through.
7. While the fish is baking, toss the asparagus with olive oil, salt, and pepper, and spread them out on a separate baking sheet.
8. Roast the asparagus in the oven for about 10-15 minutes, until they are tender and slightly browned.
9. Serve the almond-crusted cod with the roasted asparagus on the side.

Nutritional values (per serving):

Calories: 422
Total Fat: 27g
Saturated Fat: 3g
Cholesterol: 126mg
Sodium: 208mg
Total Carbohydrates: 7g
Dietary Fiber: 4g
Sugars: 1g
Protein: 39g

Octopus luciana style

Preparation Time: 30 minutes **Cooking Time:** 1 hour **Servings**: 4-6 **Difficulty:** Medium

Ingredients:

- 1 large octopus, cleaned (about 2 lbs or 1 kg)
- 1/2 cup extra-virgin olive oil
- 1 onion, chopped
- 2 garlic cloves, chopped
- 1 cup canned tomatoes, chopped
- 1/2 cup pitted black olives, sliced
- 1/2 cup dry white wine
- 1 teaspoon red pepper flakes
- Salt and pepper
- Fresh parsley, chopped

Preparation:

1. Preheat the oven to 350°F (180°C).
2. Clean the octopus by removing the beak and the eyes and washing it well.
3. In a large pot, bring water to a boil and add the octopus. Cook it for 10 minutes.
4. Drain the octopus and let it cool.
5. Cut the octopus into pieces and set aside.
6. In a large ovenproof pan, heat the olive oil over medium heat. Add the onion and garlic and sauté until soft.
7. Add the chopped tomatoes, red pepper flakes, and olives. Cook for a few minutes until the sauce thickens.
8. Add the octopus and white wine to the pan. Season with salt and pepper.
9. Cover the pan with aluminum foil and bake in the oven for 45-50 minutes.
10. Serve hot, garnished with chopped parsley.

Nutritional values (per serving):

Calories: 380
Fat: 23g
Saturated Fat: 3.5g
Cholesterol: 60mg
Sodium: 620mg

Carbohydrates: 10g
Fiber: 2g
Sugar: 4g
Protein: 30g

Stuffed Squid

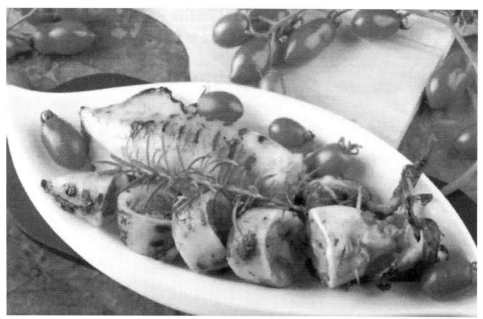

Preparation time: 20 minutes **Cooking time:** 15 minutes **Servings:** 4-5 **Difficulty:** Easy

Ingredients:

- 8-10 small to medium squid (cleaned and prepared)
- 1/2 cup cooked quinoa
- 1/2 cup chopped cherry tomatoes
- 1/4 cup chopped Kalamata olives
- 1/4 cup chopped fresh parsley
- 2 cloves garlic, minced
- 1/4 teaspoon red pepper flakes
- Salt and pepper to taste
- 1 tablespoon olive oil
- 1 lemon, cut into wedges

Preparation:

1. Preheat oven to 375°F (190°C).
2. In a medium bowl, combine quinoa, cherry tomatoes, Kalamata olives, parsley, garlic, red pepper flakes, salt, and pepper. Mix well.
3. Stuff each squid with the quinoa mixture, filling about 3/4 full. Secure the opening with toothpicks.
4. Heat olive oil in a large oven-safe skillet over medium-high heat. Add the stuffed squid and cook for 2-3 minutes per side until lightly browned.
5. Transfer the skillet to the oven and bake for 10-12 minutes, or until the squid is cooked through and tender.
6. Serve hot with lemon wedges on the side.

Nutritional values per serving (1 squid):

- Calories: 160 kcal
- Protein: 15g
- Fat: 4g
- Carbohydrates: 17g
- Fiber: 3g
- Sodium: 380mg

Baked Salmon with Lemon and Herbs

Preparation time: 10 minutes **Cooking time:** 15 minutes **Difficulty:** Easy **Portions:** 4

Ingredients:
- 4 6-oz salmon fillets
- 2 tbsp olive oil
- 2 tbsp chopped fresh parsley
- 1 tbsp chopped fresh dill
- 1 tbsp chopped fresh chives
- 1 lemon, sliced
- Salt and pepper to taste

Instructions:
1. Preheat the oven to 400°F.
2. Line a baking sheet with foil and lightly oil the foil.
3. Place the salmon fillets on the prepared baking sheet and brush each fillet with olive oil.
4. Sprinkle the chopped herbs over the fillets and place a slice of lemon on top of each one.
5. Season with salt and pepper to taste.
6. Bake for 12-15 minutes, until the salmon is cooked through and flakes easily with a fork.
7. Serve hot.

Nutritional values (per serving):
Calories: 281 Protein: 35g Carbohydrates: 1g Fat: 14g Fiber: 0g Sodium: 165mg

Salmon and Quinoa Bowl

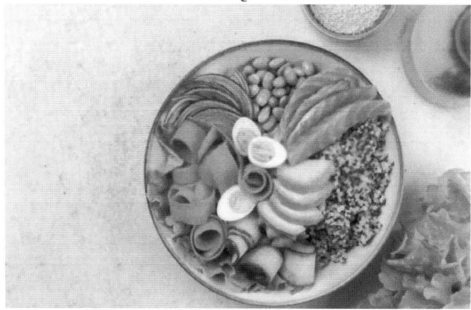

Preparation time: 10 minutes **Cooking time**: 20 minutes **Difficulty:** Easy **Portions:** 4

Ingredients:
- 1 cup quinoa, rinsed
- 2 cups low-sodium vegetable broth
- 4 (4 oz) skinless salmon fillets
- 2 tbsp olive oil
- 1 tsp dried thyme
- Salt and pepper to taste
- 4 cups baby spinach
- 1 avocado, sliced
- 1/4 cup crumbled feta cheese
- Juice of 1 lemon

Instructions:

In a medium saucepan, bring the quinoa and vegetable broth to a boil. Reduce the heat to low, cover the pan, and simmer for 15-20 minutes, until the quinoa is tender and the broth has been absorbed. Preheat the broiler. Place the salmon fillets on a baking sheet lined with parchment paper. Drizzle the salmon with olive oil and sprinkle with thyme, salt, and pepper. Broil the salmon for 10-12 minutes, until cooked through. Divide the cooked quinoa among four bowls. Top each bowl with spinach, avocado, and crumbled feta cheese. Place a salmon fillet on top of each bowl. Squeeze lemon juice over the salmon and serve.

Nutritional values per serving:
Calories: 439Protein: 32g Carbohydrates: 25g Fat: 23g Fiber: 7g Sodium: 429mg

VEGETARIAN RECIPES

Roasted Vegetable and Quinoa Salad

time: 20 minutes **Cooking time:** 25 minutes **Difficulty:** Easy **Portions:** 4

Ingredients:

- 1 cup quinoa, rinsed and drained
- 2 cups water
- 1 small eggplant, diced
- 1 red bell pepper, diced
- 1 yellow bell pepper, diced
- 1 zucchini, diced
- 1 red onion, diced
- 2 tbsp olive oil
- Salt and pepper to taste
- 1/4 cup chopped fresh parsley
- 2 tbsp lemon juice

Instructions:

1. Preheat the oven to 400°F.
2. In a medium saucepan, bring the quinoa and water to a boil over high heat.
3. Reduce the heat to low, cover the saucepan, and simmer the quinoa for 15-20 minutes, until tender and the water has been absorbed.
4. In a large bowl, toss the eggplant, red and yellow bell peppers, zucchini, and red onion with 2 tablespoons of olive oil.
5. Season the vegetables with salt and pepper to taste.
6. Spread the vegetables in a single layer on a baking sheet and roast them for 20-25 minutes, until tender and lightly browned.
7. In a small bowl, whisk together the lemon juice, 1 tablespoon of olive oil, and salt and pepper to taste.
8. In a large bowl, combine the cooked quinoa, roasted vegetables, chopped parsley, and lemon vinaigrette.
9. Toss to combine and serve at room temperature.

Nutritional values (per serving):

Calories: 291
Protein: 9g
Carbohydrates: 43g
Fat: 10g
Fiber: 8g
Sodium: 20mg

Vegetable Meatballs with Spaghetti Squash

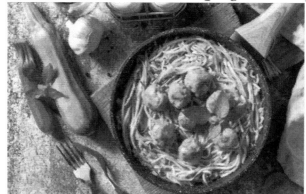

Preparation Time: 30 minutes **Cooking Time:** 1 hour **Difficulty:** Easy **Portions:** 4

Ingredients:

For the Meatballs:
- 1 can (15 ounces) chickpeas, drained and rinsed
- 1/2 cup chopped onion
- 1/2 cup shredded carrots
- 1/2 cup chopped kale
- 1/4 cup chopped fresh parsley
- 1/4 cup whole wheat breadcrumbs
- 1/4 cup grated Parmesan cheese
- 2 cloves garlic, minced
- 1 egg, beaten
- 1/2 teaspoon dried oregano
- Salt and black pepper to taste
- 2 tablespoons olive oil

For the Spaghetti Squash:
- 2 medium spaghetti squash
- 1 tablespoon olive oil
- Salt and black pepper to taste

For the Tomato Sauce:
- 1 can (14 ounces) diced tomatoes, undrained
- 2 cloves garlic, minced
- 1 tablespoon olive oil
- 1/2 teaspoon dried basil
- 1/2 teaspoon dried oregano
- Salt and black pepper to taste

Instructions:
1. Preheat the oven to 375°F (190°C).
2. Cut the spaghetti squash in half lengthwise and scoop out the seeds. Drizzle the squash halves with olive oil and sprinkle with salt and black pepper. Place the squash halves, cut side down, on a baking sheet. Bake for 40-45 minutes, or until the squash is tender and the flesh separates easily into spaghetti-like strands.
3. While the spaghetti squash is baking, prepare the meatballs. In a food processor, pulse the chickpeas until they are finely chopped. Transfer the chickpeas to a large bowl.
4. Add the onion, carrots, kale, parsley, breadcrumbs, Parmesan cheese, garlic, egg, oregano, salt, and black pepper to the bowl with the chickpeas. Mix well to combine.
5. Using a tablespoon, scoop out the mixture and shape it into balls, making 20-24 meatballs.
6. Heat the olive oil in a large skillet over medium heat. Add the meatballs and cook for 15-20 minutes, or until golden brown and cooked through.
7. While the meatballs are cooking, prepare the tomato sauce. In a small saucepan, heat the olive oil over medium heat. Add the garlic and cook for 1-2 minutes, or until fragrant. Add the diced tomatoes, basil, oregano, salt, and black pepper. Simmer for 10-15 minutes, or until the sauce is slightly thickened.
8. To serve, spoon the tomato sauce over the spaghetti squash and top with the vegetable meatballs.

Nutritional Information per serving:
Calories: 399

Fat: 16g

Saturated Fat: 3g

Cholesterol: 53mg

Sodium: 624mg

Carbohydrates: 49g

Fiber: 13g

Sugar: 13g

Chickpea Burgers

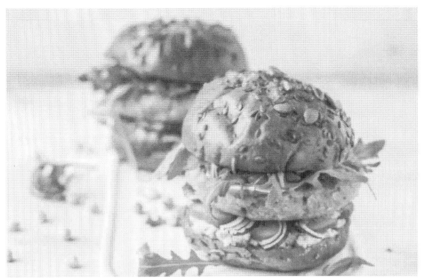

Preparation Time: 20 minutes **Cooking Time:** 15 minutes **Difficulty:** Easy **Portions:** 4

Ingredients:

- 2 cans (15 ounces each) chickpeas, drained and rinsed
- 1/2 cup chopped onion
- 1/2 cup chopped mushrooms
- 1/2 cup chopped carrots
- 1/2 cup chopped parsley
- 1/2 cup whole wheat breadcrumbs
- 1/4 cup grated Parmesan cheese
- 2 cloves garlic, minced
- 1 egg, beaten
- 1 teaspoon ground cumin
- 1/2 teaspoon paprika
- Salt and black pepper to taste
- 2 tablespoons olive oil

For serving:

- 4 whole wheat burger buns
- 4 lettuce leaves
- 4 tomato slices
- 4 tablespoons low-fat plain Greek yogurt
- 4 tablespoons mustard

Instructions:

1. In a food processor, pulse the chickpeas until they are finely chopped. Transfer the chickpeas to a large bowl.
2. Add the onion, mushrooms, carrots, parsley, breadcrumbs, Parmesan cheese, garlic, egg, cumin, paprika, salt, and black pepper to the bowl with the chickpeas. Mix well to combine.
3. Using a 1/2 cup measuring cup, scoop out the mixture and shape it into patties, making 8 patties.
4. Heat the olive oil in a large skillet over medium heat. Add the patties and cook for 7-8 minutes on each side, or until golden brown and cooked through.
5. To serve, place a lettuce leaf and a tomato slice on the bottom half of each bun. Top with a chickpea patty, a tablespoon of Greek yogurt, and a tablespoon of mustard. Cover with the top half of the bun.

Nutritional Information per serving:

Calories: 423

Fat: 13g

Saturated Fat: 2g

Cholesterol: 53mg

Sodium: 871mg

Carbohydrates: 63g

Fiber: 16g

Sugar: 12g

Protein: 22

White Zucchini Parmigiana

Preparation Time: 15 minutes **Cooking Time**: 45 minutes **Difficulty**: Easy **Portions**: 4

Ingredients:

- 4 medium zucchini, sliced lengthwise
- 1/4 cup all-purpose flour
- 1/4 cup grated Parmesan cheese
- 1/2 teaspoon garlic powder
- Salt and black pepper to taste
- 2 tablespoons olive oil
- 2 cups marinara sauce
- 1 cup part-skim ricotta cheese
- 1 cup shredded part-skim mozzarella cheese
- 1/4 cup chopped fresh basil

Instructions:

1. Preheat the oven to 375°F (190°C).
2. In a shallow dish, mix the flour, Parmesan cheese, garlic powder, salt, and black pepper.
3. Dip each zucchini slice into the flour mixture to coat.
4. Heat the olive oil in a large skillet over medium heat. Add the zucchini slices and cook for 2-3 minutes on each side, or until lightly browned.
5. Spread 1/2 cup of the marinara sauce in the bottom of an 8x8-inch baking dish. Layer half of the zucchini slices on top of the sauce.
6. In a bowl, mix the ricotta cheese, 1/2 cup of the mozzarella cheese, and half of the chopped basil. Spread this mixture on top of the zucchini slices in the baking dish.
7. Layer the remaining zucchini slices on top of the cheese mixture. Pour the remaining marinara sauce over the zucchini slices.
8. Top with the remaining 1/2 cup of mozzarella cheese.
9. Bake for 30-35 minutes, or until the cheese is melted and bubbly and the zucchini is tender.
10. Let cool for a few minutes before serving. Garnish with the remaining chopped basil.

Nutritional Information per serving: Calories: 300 Fat: 16g Saturated Fat: 7g Cholesterol: 39mg Sodium: 834mg Carbohydrates: 18g Fiber: 4g Sugar: 9g Protein: 21g

Cabbage Rolls with Baked Potatoes

Preparation Time: 30 minutes **Cooking Time**: 1 hour **Difficulty**: Medium **Portions**: 4

Ingredients:

For the Cabbage Rolls:

- 1 large head of cabbage
- 1 cup cooked rice
- 1 onion, finely chopped
- 2 garlic cloves, minced
- 1/2 teaspoon paprika
- 1/2 teaspoon dried oregano
- Salt and black pepper to taste
- 1 can (15 oz) tomato sauce
- 1/2 cup vegetable broth
- 1/4 cup chopped fresh parsley

For the Baked Potatoes:

- 4 large potatoes, scrubbed and pierced with a fork
- 2 tablespoons olive oil
- Salt and black pepper to taste

Instructions:

1. Preheat the oven to 375°F.
2. Bring a large pot of water to a boil. Add the head of cabbage and cook for 5-7 minutes, or until the leaves are pliable. Remove the cabbage from the pot and let it cool. Once cooled, carefully remove the leaves one by one and set them aside.
3. In a large bowl, combine the cooked rice, onion, garlic, paprika, oregano, salt, and black pepper. Mix well.
4. Take one cabbage leaf and place 1-2 tablespoons of the rice mixture in the center. Fold the sides of the cabbage leaf over the filling and roll up to create a tight package. Repeat with the remaining cabbage leaves and filling.

5. In a large baking dish, combine the tomato sauce and vegetable broth. Place the cabbage rolls on top of the tomato sauce mixture. Cover the dish with foil and bake for 45-50 minutes, or until the cabbage rolls are cooked through.
6. While the cabbage rolls are cooking, prepare the baked potatoes. Rub the potatoes with olive oil and sprinkle with salt and black pepper. Place the potatoes on a baking sheet and bake for 45-50 minutes, or until tender.
7. Serve the cabbage rolls with the tomato sauce and chopped fresh parsley. Serve the baked potatoes on the side.

Nutritional Information per serving: Calories:401 Fat:9g Saturated Fat:1g Cholesterol:0mg Sodium:807mg Carbohydrates:75g Fiber:11g Sugar:14g Protein:9g

Cauliflower Casserole

Preparation Time: 15 minutes **Cooking Time:** 40 minutes **Difficulty:** Easy **Portions:** 4-6
Ingredients:
- 1 large head of cauliflower, cut into florets
- 1 tablespoon olive oil
- 1 onion, chopped
- 2 garlic cloves, minced
- 1 can (15 oz) diced tomatoes
- 1 teaspoon dried basil
- 1 teaspoon dried oregano
- Salt and black pepper to taste
- 1 cup shredded mozzarella cheese
- 1/4 cup grated Parmesan cheese

Instructions:
1. Preheat the oven to 375°F.
2. Steam the cauliflower florets for 5-7 minutes, or until they are tender but still slightly firm. Drain and set aside.
3. In a large skillet, heat the olive oil over medium heat. Add the onion and garlic and cook for 3-4 minutes, or until softened.
4. Add the diced tomatoes, basil, oregano, salt, and black pepper to the skillet. Stir to combine and cook for 5-7 minutes, or until the sauce has thickened slightly.
5. Add the cauliflower to the skillet and stir to coat with the tomato sauce.
6. Transfer the cauliflower mixture to a large baking dish. Sprinkle the shredded mozzarella cheese and grated Parmesan cheese on top.
7. Bake for 25-30 minutes, or until the cheese is melted and bubbly and the casserole is heated through.
8. Let the casserole cool for a few minutes before serving.

Nutritional Information per serving (based on 6 servings):
Calories: 158 Fat:9g Saturated Fat: 4g Cholesterol:22mg Sodium:441mg Carbohydrates:10g Fiber:3g Sugar:5g Protein:12g

Beetroot Savory Pie

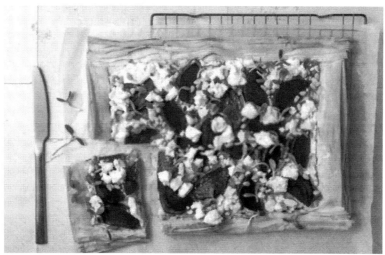

Preparation Time: 30 minutes **Cooking Time:** 45 minutes **Difficulty**: Medium **Portions**: 6-8

Ingredients:

For the crust:

- 1 1/2 cups whole wheat flour
- 1/2 cup cornmeal
- 1/2 teaspoon salt
- 1/2 cup cold unsalted butter, cut into small cubes
- 1/4 cup ice water

For the filling:

- 1 large beetroot, peeled and diced
- 2 tablespoons olive oil
- 1 onion, chopped
- 2 garlic cloves, minced
- 1/4 teaspoon dried thyme
- 1/4 teaspoon dried rosemary
- Salt and black pepper to taste
- 2 cups fresh spinach leaves, chopped
- 1/2 cup crumbled feta cheese
- 2 eggs
- 1/2 cup skim milk

Instructions:

1. Preheat the oven to 375°F.
2. In a large mixing bowl, whisk together the flour, cornmeal, and salt.
3. Add the butter cubes to the bowl and use a pastry blender or your fingers to cut the butter into the flour mixture until it resembles coarse crumbs.
4. Gradually add the ice water to the bowl, a tablespoon at a time, until the dough comes together into a ball.
5. On a lightly floured surface, roll out the dough into a large circle that will fit into a 9-inch pie dish. Place the dough into the pie dish and trim the edges as necessary.
6. In a large skillet, heat the olive oil over medium heat. Add the onion and garlic and cook for 3-4 minutes, or until softened.
7. Add the diced beetroot, thyme, rosemary, salt, and black pepper to the skillet. Stir to combine and cook for 5-7 minutes, or until the beetroot is tender.
8. Add the chopped spinach to the skillet and cook for 2-3 minutes, or until the spinach is wilted.
9. In a mixing bowl, whisk together the eggs and skim milk. Add the feta cheese to the bowl and stir to combine.
10. Add the cooked beetroot and spinach mixture to the pie crust in the dish. Pour the egg and milk mixture over the vegetables.
11. Bake for 35-40 minutes, or until the pie is set and the crust is golden brown.

Nutritional Information per serving (based on 8 servings):

Calories: 280 Fat: 15g Saturated Fat: 8g Cholesterol: 84mg Sodium: 340mg Carbohydrates: 25g Fiber: 4g Sugar: 3g Protein: 10g

Kale Burgers

Preparation Time: 30 minutes **Cooking Time**: 20 minutes **Difficulty:** Medium Portions: 4

Ingredients:

- 1 can (15 oz) chickpeas, drained and rinsed
- 1/2 cup chopped kale
- 1/4 cup chopped onion
- 2 cloves garlic, minced
- 1 tablespoon lemon juice
- 1/2 teaspoon cumin
- 1/2 teaspoon paprika
- 1/4 teaspoon salt
- 1/4 teaspoon black pepper
- 1/4 cup breadcrumbs
- 1/4 cup grated Parmesan cheese
- 1 large egg, lightly beaten
- 4 whole wheat hamburger buns
- Toppings of your choice (lettuce, tomato, avocado, etc.)

Instructions:

1. Preheat the oven to 375°F.
2. In a food processor, pulse the chickpeas, kale, onion, garlic, lemon juice, cumin, paprika, salt, and black pepper until well combined.
3. Transfer the mixture to a mixing bowl and stir in the breadcrumbs, Parmesan cheese, and egg.
4. Form the mixture into 4 equal-sized patties.
5. Heat a nonstick skillet over medium heat. Add the patties and cook for 3-4 minutes per side, or until golden brown.
6. Transfer the patties to a baking sheet and bake in the oven for 10-12 minutes, or until heated through.
7. Serve the patties on whole wheat hamburger buns with your favorite toppings.

Nutritional Information per serving:

Calories: 310 Fat: 8g Saturated Fat: 2.5g Cholesterol: 65mg Sodium: 610mg Carbohydrates: 45g Fiber: 10g Sugar: 5g Protein: 16g

Rustic potato and onion pie

Preparation Time: 20 minutes **Cooking Time:** 50 minutes **Difficulty:** Easy **Portions:** 6

Ingredients:

- 2 large potatoes, peeled and sliced
- 1 large onion, sliced
- 1 tablespoon olive oil
- 2 cloves garlic, minced
- 1/2 teaspoon dried thyme
- 1/4 teaspoon salt
- 1/4 teaspoon black pepper
- 1/2 cup vegetable broth
- 1 refrigerated pie crust
- 1 egg, lightly beaten

Instructions:

1. Preheat the oven to 375°F.
2. In a large skillet, heat the olive oil over medium heat. Add the sliced potatoes, onion, garlic, thyme, salt, and black pepper. Cook for 8-10 minutes, or until the potatoes are tender and the onion is translucent.
3. Add the vegetable broth to the skillet and bring to a simmer. Cook for 2-3 minutes, or until the liquid has reduced and thickened slightly.
4. Roll out the pie crust and place it in a 9-inch pie dish. Trim the edges.
5. Spoon the potato mixture into the pie crust.
6. Brush the edges of the pie crust with the beaten egg.
7. Bake in the oven for 30-35 minutes, or until the crust is golden brown and the filling is heated through.
8. Let cool for a few minutes before serving.

Nutritional Information per serving:

Calories: 220 Fat: 10g Saturated Fat: 2.5g Cholesterol: 25mg Sodium: 390mg Carbohydrates: 28g Fiber: 2g Sugar: 2g Protein: 4g

Spinach Cutlets

Preparation Time: 20 minutes **Cooking Time**: 25 minutes **Difficulty:** Easy **Portions:** 4

Ingredients:

- 2 cups chopped spinach
- 1/2 cup crumbled paneer (Indian cheese) or tofu
- 1/2 cup mashed potatoes
- 1/2 cup bread crumbs
- 1/4 cup chopped onion
- 2 cloves garlic, minced
- 1 green chili pepper, finely chopped
- 1/2 teaspoon ground cumin
- 1/2 teaspoon ground coriander
- 1/4 teaspoon garam masala (Indian spice blend)
- Salt and black pepper to taste
- 2 tablespoons vegetable oil

Instructions:

1. In a large mixing bowl, combine the chopped spinach, crumbled paneer or tofu, mashed potatoes, bread crumbs, chopped onion, minced garlic, finely chopped green chili pepper, ground cumin, ground coriander, garam masala, salt, and black pepper. Mix well.
2. Shape the mixture into small patties or cutlets.
3. Heat the vegetable oil in a large skillet over medium heat.
4. Place the patties or cutlets in the skillet and cook until golden brown on both sides, about 3-4 minutes per side.
5. Serve hot with chutney or sauce of your choice.

Nutritional Information per serving:

Calories: 245 Fat: 13g Saturated Fat: 2g Cholesterol: 5mg Sodium: 388mg Carbohydrates: 25g Fiber: 3g Sugar: 3g Protein: 8g

Lentil and potato meatballs with gravy

Preparation Time: 20 minutes **Cooking Time:** 45 minutes **Difficulty:** Medium **Portions**: 4

Ingredients:

For the Meatballs:

- 1 cup cooked lentils, drained
- 1 cup boiled potatoes, mashed
- 1/2 cup bread crumbs
- 1/4 cup finely chopped onion
- 2 cloves garlic, minced
- 2 tablespoons chopped fresh parsley
- 1 tablespoon chopped fresh thyme
- 1/2 teaspoon ground cumin
- Salt and black pepper to taste
- 1 tablespoon vegetable oil

For the Gravy:

- 2 tablespoons vegetable oil
- 2 tablespoons all-purpose flour
- 2 cups vegetable broth
- 1/2 teaspoon dried thyme
- Salt and black pepper to taste

Instructions:

1. Preheat the oven to 375°F (190°C).
2. In a large mixing bowl, combine the cooked lentils, mashed potatoes, bread crumbs, finely chopped onion, minced garlic, chopped fresh parsley, chopped fresh thyme, ground cumin, salt, and black pepper. Mix well.
3. Shape the mixture into small balls and place them on a baking sheet lined with parchment paper.
4. Drizzle the meatballs with vegetable oil and bake for 25-30 minutes, or until golden brown.
5. Meanwhile, prepare the gravy. Heat the vegetable oil in a saucepan over medium heat.
6. Add the all-purpose flour and whisk until combined. Cook for 1-2 minutes, or until the mixture turns golden brown.
7. Slowly pour in the vegetable broth, whisking constantly to avoid lumps. Add the dried thyme, salt, and black pepper. Bring to a boil, then reduce the heat and simmer for 10-15 minutes, or until the gravy thickens.
8. Serve the meatballs hot, topped with the gravy.

Quinoa-Stuffed Bell Peppers

Preparation Time: 20 minutes **Cooking Time:** 1 hour **Difficulty:** Easy **Portions:** 4

Ingredients:

- 4 large bell peppers, any color
- 1 cup quinoa, rinsed and drained
- 1 3/4 cups vegetable broth
- 1 can (14 ounces) diced tomatoes, undrained
- 1 can (15 ounces) black beans, rinsed and drained
- 1/2 cup frozen corn
- 1/2 cup diced onion
- 1/2 cup diced red bell pepper
- 1/2 cup shredded cheddar cheese
- 1 tablespoon olive oil
- 1 teaspoon chili powder
- 1/2 teaspoon cumin
- Salt and black pepper to taste

Instructions:

1. Preheat the oven to 375°F (190°C). Grease a large baking dish.
2. Cut off the tops of the bell peppers and remove the seeds and membranes.
3. In a large saucepan, bring the quinoa and vegetable broth to a boil. Reduce the heat, cover the saucepan, and simmer for 15-20 minutes, or until the quinoa is tender and the broth is absorbed.
4. In a large skillet, heat the olive oil over medium heat. Add the onion and red bell pepper and cook until softened, about 5-7 minutes.
5. Add the diced tomatoes, black beans, corn, chili powder, cumin, salt, and black pepper to the skillet. Cook for 5-7 minutes, or until the vegetables are tender and the mixture is heated through.
6. Stir the cooked quinoa into the skillet mixture.
7. Stuff the bell peppers with the quinoa mixture and place them in the prepared baking dish. Top each bell pepper with a sprinkle of shredded cheese.
8. Bake for 25-30 minutes, or until the bell peppers are tender and the cheese is melted and bubbly.

Nutritional Information per serving:

Calories: 364 Fat: 10g Saturated Fat: 3g Cholesterol: 13mg Sodium: 792mg Carbohydrates: 55g Fiber: 13g Sugar: 12g Protein: 18g

VEGAN RECIPES

Bean Meatballs

Preparation Time: 20 minutes **Cooking Time:** 25 minutes **Difficulty:** Easy **Servings:** 4

Ingredients:

For the meatballs:

- 1 can (15 ounces) chickpeas, drained and rinsed
- 1/2 cup bread crumbs
- 1/4 cup nutritional yeast
- 1/4 cup finely chopped onion
- 2 cloves garlic, minced
- 2 tablespoons chopped fresh parsley
- 1 teaspoon dried oregano
- 1/2 teaspoon smoked paprika
- Salt and pepper, to taste
- 1 tablespoon ground flaxseed mixed with 3 tablespoons water (flaxseed egg)
- 2 tablespoons olive oil, for cooking

For the tomato sauce:

- 1 can (14 ounces) crushed tomatoes
- 1 clove garlic, minced
- 1/2 teaspoon dried basil
- 1/2 teaspoon dried oregano
- Salt and pepper, to taste

Instructions:

1. Preheat the oven to 375°F (190°C) and line a baking sheet with parchment paper.
2. In a food processor, combine the drained and rinsed chickpeas, bread crumbs, nutritional yeast, chopped onion, minced garlic, parsley, dried oregano, smoked paprika, salt, and pepper. Pulse until well combined but still slightly chunky.
3. Transfer the mixture to a bowl and add the flaxseed egg. Mix well until the mixture holds together. If it feels too dry, you can add a tablespoon of water at a time until the desired consistency is reached.
4. Shape the mixture into small meatballs, about 1 inch in diameter, and place them on the prepared baking sheet.
5. Bake the meatballs in the preheated oven for 20-25 minutes, or until they are golden brown and firm.
6. While the meatballs are baking, prepare the tomato sauce. In a saucepan, combine the crushed tomatoes, minced garlic, dried basil, dried oregano, salt, and pepper. Cook over medium heat for about 10 minutes, stirring occasionally.
7. Once the meatballs are cooked, remove them from the oven and gently toss them in the tomato sauce until coated.
8. Serve the vegan bean meatballs with the tomato sauce over pasta, rice, or as a sandwich filling. Garnish with fresh herbs, if desired.
9.

Nutritional Information (per serving):

Calories: 285

Fat: 10g

Saturated Fat: 1g

Trans Fat: 0g

Cholesterol: 0mg

Sodium: 594mg

Carbohydrates: 36g

Fiber: 8g

Sugar: 6g

Protein: 12

Fried Tofu

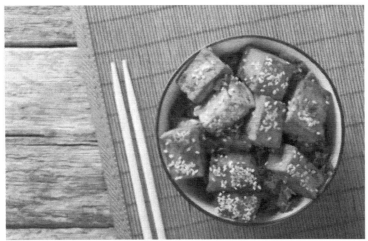

Preparation Time: 10 minutes **Cooking Time:** 15 minutes **Difficulty:** Easy **Servings:** 4

Ingredients:

- 1 block (14 ounces) firm tofu
- 1/2 cup cornstarch
- 1 teaspoon garlic powder
- 1 teaspoon paprika
- 1/2 teaspoon salt
- 1/4 teaspoon black pepper
- Vegetable oil, for frying

For the dipping sauce:

- 2 tablespoons soy sauce
- 1 tablespoon rice vinegar
- 1 tablespoon maple syrup
- 1/2 teaspoon sesame oil
- 1/2 teaspoon grated ginger
- Sesame seeds, for garnish (optional)
- Chopped green onions, for garnish (optional)

Instructions:

1. Press the tofu: Start by pressing the tofu to remove excess moisture. Place the tofu block on a plate lined with paper towels or a clean kitchen towel. Put another layer of paper towels or kitchen towel on top of the tofu. Place a heavy object, such as a cutting board or a can of beans, on top of the towel to weigh it down. Let it sit for about 15 minutes to remove the water.
2. Cut the tofu: After pressing, cut the tofu into bite-sized cubes or rectangles, depending on your preference.
3. Prepare the coating mixture: In a shallow bowl, whisk together the cornstarch, garlic powder, paprika, salt, and black pepper.
4. Coat the tofu: Roll each tofu piece in the coating mixture until fully coated. Shake off any excess coating.
5. Fry the tofu: In a large skillet, heat vegetable oil over medium heat. Add the coated tofu pieces in a single layer and fry until golden brown and crispy, about 2-3 minutes per side. Work in batches if necessary, ensuring not to overcrowd the pan.
6. Transfer the fried tofu to a paper towel-lined plate to remove any excess oil.
7. Prepare the dipping sauce: In a small bowl, whisk together the soy sauce, rice vinegar, maple syrup, sesame oil, and grated ginger until well combined.
8. Serve the vegan fried tofu hot, with the dipping sauce on the side. Garnish with sesame seeds and chopped green onions, if desired.

Nutritional Information (per serving):

Calories: 228
Fat: 11g
Saturated Fat: 1g
Trans Fat: 0g
Cholesterol: 0mg

Sodium: 634mg
Carbohydrates: 24g
Fiber: 1g
Sugar: 4g
Protein: 10g

Vegan Lasagne

Preparation Time: 30 minutes **Cooking Time**: 45 minutes **Difficulty**: Medium **Servings**: 8

Ingredients:

For the tomato sauce:
- 1 tablespoon olive oil
- 1 large onion, chopped
- 3 cloves garlic, minced
- 1 can (14 ounces) crushed tomatoes
- 1 can (14 ounces) tomato sauce
- 1 can (6 ounces) tomato paste
- 2 teaspoons dried basil
- 2 teaspoons dried oregano
- 1 teaspoon sugar (optional)
- Salt and pepper, to taste

For the tofu ricotta:
- 1 block (14 ounces) firm tofu, drained
- 2 tablespoons nutritional yeast
- 2 tablespoons lemon juice
- 2 cloves garlic, minced
- 1 teaspoon dried basil
- 1 teaspoon dried oregano
- Salt and pepper, to taste

Other ingredients:
- 9 lasagne noodles, cooked according to package instructions
- 3 cups fresh spinach leaves
- 2 cups sliced mushrooms
- 2 cups shredded vegan mozzarella cheese
- Fresh basil leaves, for garnish (optional)

Instructions:

1. Preheat the oven to 375°F (190°C).
2. Prepare the tomato sauce: In a large saucepan, heat the olive oil over medium heat. Add the chopped onion and minced garlic, and sauté until the onion becomes translucent.
3. Add the crushed tomatoes, tomato sauce, tomato paste, dried basil, dried oregano, sugar (if using), salt, and pepper to the saucepan. Stir well to combine. Simmer the sauce for about 15-20 minutes, allowing the flavors to meld together. Adjust the seasonings to taste.
4. Prepare the tofu ricotta: In a mixing bowl, crumble the drained tofu with your hands or a fork until it resembles ricotta cheese. Add the nutritional yeast, lemon juice, minced garlic, dried basil, dried oregano, salt, and pepper. Mix well to combine.
5. Assemble the lasagne: Spread a thin layer of the tomato sauce on the bottom of a 9x13-inch baking dish. Arrange 3 cooked lasagne noodles on top of the sauce. Spread half of the tofu ricotta mixture over the noodles, followed by half of the spinach and mushrooms. Pour about 1 cup of tomato sauce over the vegetables.
6. Repeat the layering process with 3 more lasagne noodles, the remaining tofu ricotta mixture, the remaining spinach and mushrooms, and another cup of tomato sauce.
7. Place the final 3 lasagne noodles on top and cover them with the remaining tomato sauce. Sprinkle the shredded vegan mozzarella cheese evenly over the top.
8. Cover the baking dish with foil and bake in the preheated oven for 25 minutes. Remove the foil and bake for an additional 10 minutes, or until the cheese is melted and bubbly.
9. Once baked, remove the lasagne from the oven and let it cool for a few minutes. Garnish with fresh basil leaves, if desired.

Nutritional Information (per serving):

Calories: 367
Fat: 9g
Saturated Fat: 1g
Trans Fat: 0g
Cholesterol: 0mg

Sodium: 487mg
Carbohydrates: 51g
Fiber: 7g
Sugar: 9g
Protein: 23g

Vegan Pasta with Pesto and Celery Leaves

Preparation Time: 15 minutes **Cooking Time:** 10 minutes **Difficulty:** Easy **Portions:** 4 servings

Ingredients:

- 8 ounces whole wheat pasta
- 2 cups fresh basil leaves
- 1/4 cup walnuts
- 2 cloves garlic, minced
- 1/4 cup nutritional yeast
- 2 tablespoons lemon juice
- 1/4 cup extra virgin olive oil
- 1/2 teaspoon salt
- 1/4 teaspoon black pepper
- 1 cup celery leaves, chopped
- 1 cup cherry tomatoes, halved

Instructions:

1. Cook the whole wheat pasta according to the package instructions until al dente. Drain and set aside.
2. In a food processor, combine the fresh basil leaves, walnuts, minced garlic, nutritional yeast, lemon juice, olive oil, salt, and black pepper. Process until well blended and smooth.
3. In a large mixing bowl, combine the cooked pasta, pesto sauce, chopped celery leaves, and cherry tomatoes. Toss well to coat the pasta evenly with the sauce.
4. Let the pasta sit for a few minutes to allow the flavors to meld together.
5. Serve the pasta warm or at room temperature, garnished with additional basil leaves if desired.

Nutritional Values (per serving):

Calories: 350 kcal

Carbohydrates: 45g

Protein: 10g

Fat: 16g

Fiber: 8g

Sugar: 3g

Sodium: 280mg

Rice with Seitan Ragu

Preparation Time: 15 minutes **Cooking Time:** 45 minutes **Difficulty:** Medium **Servings:** 4

Ingredients:

For the seitan ragu:

- 2 tablespoons olive oil
- 1 medium onion, finely chopped
- 2 cloves garlic, minced
- 1 green bell pepper, finely chopped
- 1 carrot, finely chopped
- 8 ounces seitan, chopped into small pieces
- 1 can (14 ounces) crushed tomatoes
- 1 can (6 ounces) tomato paste
- 1 teaspoon dried basil
- 1 teaspoon dried oregano
- 1/2 teaspoon sugar
- Salt and pepper, to taste

For the rice:

- 1 cup long-grain white rice
- 2 cups vegetable broth
- 1 tablespoon olive oil

For garnish:

- Fresh parsley, chopped

Instructions:

1. In a large saucepan, heat the olive oil over medium heat. Add the chopped onion and minced garlic, and sauté until the onion becomes translucent.
2. Add the chopped green bell pepper and carrot to the saucepan, and cook for another 2-3 minutes until the vegetables begin to soften.
3. Add the seitan to the saucepan and cook for 5 minutes, stirring occasionally.
4. Stir in the crushed tomatoes, tomato paste, dried basil, dried oregano, sugar, salt, and pepper. Reduce the heat to low, cover, and simmer for 30 minutes, allowing the flavors to meld together. Adjust the seasonings to taste.
5. While the ragu is simmering, prepare the rice. In a separate saucepan, heat the olive oil over medium heat. Add the rice and cook for 1-2 minutes, stirring constantly.
6. Pour in the vegetable broth and bring to a boil. Reduce the heat to low, cover, and simmer for about 15-20 minutes, or until the rice is tender and all the liquid is absorbed.
7. Once the rice is cooked, fluff it with a fork and remove it from the heat.
8. Serve the rice with a generous scoop of the seitan ragu on top. Garnish with fresh chopped parsley.

Nutritional Information (per serving):
Calories: 412

Fat: 11g

Saturated Fat: 1g

Trans Fat: 0g

Cholesterol: 0mg

Sodium: 638mg

Carbohydrates: 59g

Fiber: 6g

Sugar: 10g

Protein: 19g

SOUPS
Spicy Thai coconut soup

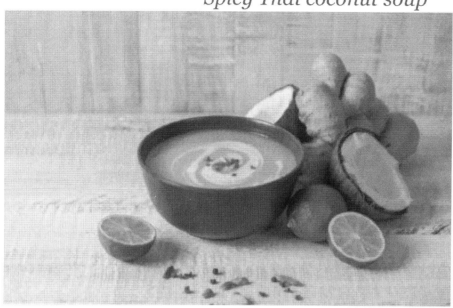

Preparation Time: 10 minutes **Cooking Time:** 25 minutes **Difficulty:** Easy **Portions:** 4

Ingredients:

- 1 tablespoon olive oil
- 1 onion, chopped
- 2 garlic cloves, minced
- 1 tablespoon ginger, minced
- 1 red bell pepper, chopped
- 1 green bell pepper, chopped
- 2 tablespoons red curry paste
- 4 cups low-sodium chicken or vegetable broth
- 1 can (14 oz) light coconut milk
- 1 pound skinless, boneless chicken breast, cubed

- **1 lime, juiced**
- **1 tablespoon fish sauce**
- **1 tablespoon low-sodium soy sauce**
- **1 tablespoon brown sugar**
- **1/4 teaspoon salt**
- **1/4 teaspoon black pepper**
- **2 tablespoons fresh cilantro, chopped**
- **1/4 cup scallions, chopped**
- **1/4 cup unsalted peanuts, chopped**
- **2 cups baby spinach**

Instructions:

1. In a large pot or Dutch oven, heat the olive oil over medium-high heat. Add the onion, garlic, and ginger and sauté for 2-3 minutes until softened.
2. Add the red and green bell peppers and cook for another 2-3 minutes until they start to soften.
3. Add the red curry paste and stir to combine. Cook for 1 minute until fragrant.
4. Add the chicken or vegetable broth, coconut milk, chicken breast, lime juice, fish sauce, soy sauce, brown sugar, salt, and black pepper. Bring to a boil, then reduce heat to low and let simmer for 15 minutes until chicken is cooked through.
5. Add the chopped cilantro, scallions, and chopped peanuts to the soup and stir to combine.
6. Add the baby spinach and stir until it wilts, about 1-2 minutes.
7. Serve hot and enjoy!

Nutritional Information (per serving):

Calories: 327

Fat: 14g

Saturated Fat: 6g

Sodium: 675mg

Protein: 32g

Carbohydrates: 19g

Fiber: 4g

Sugar: 8g

Clam soup

reparation time: 15 minutes **Cooking time:** 30 minutes **Difficulty:** Easy **Portions:** 6

Ingredients:

- 2 tbsp unsalted butter
- 1 onion, chopped
- 2 celery stalks, chopped
- 2 medium potatoes, peeled and diced
- 2 cups low-sodium chicken broth
- 1 cup skim milk
- 1/2 cup clam juice
- 2 cans minced clams, drained
- 1 bay leaf
- 1/2 tsp dried thyme
- 1/4 tsp salt
- 1/4 tsp black pepper
- 2 tbsp chopped fresh parsley

Instructions:

1. In a large pot, melt the butter over medium heat. Add the onion and celery, and cook until softened, about 5 minutes.
2. Add the potatoes and chicken broth to the pot, and bring to a boil. Reduce the heat and simmer for about 10 minutes, or until the potatoes are tender.
3. Add the milk, clam juice, minced clams, bay leaf, thyme, salt, and black pepper to the pot, and stir to combine.
4. Simmer the soup for another 10 minutes, or until heated through.
5. Remove the bay leaf from the soup, and ladle into bowls. Sprinkle with fresh parsley and serve hot.

Nutrition per serving:

Calories: 280

Total fat: 12g

Saturated fat: 5g

Trans fat: 0g

Cholesterol: 50mg

Sodium: 600mg

Total carbohydrate: 27g

Dietary fiber: 3g

Sugars: 4g

Protein: 17g

Vitamin D: 1mcg

Calcium: 120mg

Iron: 4mg

Potassium: 520mg

Corn soup

Ingredients:

- 4 ears of fresh corn, shucked
- 1 tbsp olive oil
- 1 onion, chopped
- 2 cloves garlic, minced
- 1 red bell pepper, chopped
- 1 small zucchini, chopped
- 4 cups low-sodium vegetable or chicken broth
- 1/2 cup low-fat or fat-free milk
- 1/4 tsp black pepper
- Salt, to taste
- Fresh cilantro or parsley, chopped, for garnish (optional)

Instructions:

1. Cut the kernels off the corn cobs and set aside. Place the cobs in a large pot and cover with water. Bring to a boil and then reduce the heat to low. Simmer for 30 minutes to make a corn broth.
2. While the broth is simmering, heat the olive oil in a large skillet over medium heat. Add the onion and garlic and cook until the onion is translucent, about 5 minutes.
3. Add the bell pepper and zucchini and cook for an additional 5 minutes.

4. Remove the cobs from the pot and discard. Add the corn kernels, vegetable or chicken broth, and black pepper to the pot. Bring to a boil and then reduce the heat to low. Simmer for 15-20 minutes, or until the vegetables are tender.
5. Use an immersion blender or transfer the soup to a blender in batches and blend until smooth.
6. Return the soup to the pot and stir in the milk. Heat through but do not boil.
7. Add salt to taste. Serve hot, garnished with fresh cilantro or parsley if desired.

Preparation time: 15 minutes **Cooking time:** 1 hour **Difficulty:** Easy **Portions:** 4
Nutritional Information per serving: Calories: 150 Total Fat: 3.5g Saturated Fat: 0.5g Cholesterol: 5mg Sodium: 100mg Total Carbohydrates: 27g Dietary Fiber: 4g Sugars: 10g Protein: 6g

Creamy Mushroom Soup

Preparation time: 10 minutes **Cooking time:** 25 minutes **Difficulty:** Easy **Portions:** 4
Ingredients:

- 1 tbsp unsalted butter
- 1 onion, chopped
- 2 garlic cloves, minced
- 1 lb mushrooms, sliced
- 4 cups low-sodium chicken or vegetable broth
- 1/2 tsp dried thyme
- 1/4 tsp salt
- 1/4 tsp black pepper
- 1/2 cup fat-free sour cream
- 2 tbsp chopped fresh parsley

Instructions:

1. In a large pot, melt the butter over medium heat. Add the onion and garlic, and cook until softened, about 5 minutes.
2. Add the mushrooms to the pot, and cook until softened and browned, about 10 minutes.
3. Add the chicken or vegetable broth, thyme, salt, and black pepper to the pot, and bring to a boil. Reduce the heat and simmer for about 10 minutes, or until heated through.
4. Remove the pot from the heat, and stir in the sour cream.
5. Ladle into bowls and sprinkle with fresh parsley. Serve hot.

Calories: 180

Total fat: 8g

Saturated fat: 2g

Trans fat: 0g

Cholesterol: 5mg

Sodium: 450mg

Total carbohydrate: 22g

Dietary fiber: 4g

Sugars: 7g

Protein: 9g

Vitamin D: 0mcg

Calcium: 110mg

Iron: 2mg

Potassium: 590mg

Carrot and turmeric soup

Preparation time: 10 minutes **Cooking time:** 30 minutes **Difficulty:** Easy **Portions:** 4
Ingredients:

- 1 tablespoon olive oil
- 1 onion, chopped
- 2 garlic cloves, minced
- 1 teaspoon grated ginger
- 1 teaspoon ground turmeric
- 1/2 teaspoon ground cumin
- 1/2 teaspoon ground coriander
- 6 cups low-sodium vegetable broth
- 1 lb carrots, peeled and chopped
- 1/2 teaspoon salt
- 1/4 teaspoon black pepper
- 1/2 cup plain Greek yogurt
- 2 tablespoons chopped fresh cilantro

Instructions:

1. Heat the olive oil in a large pot over medium heat. Add the onion and garlic and sauté until softened, about 5 minutes.
2. Add the grated ginger, turmeric, cumin, and coriander and stir to combine. Cook for 1-2 minutes until fragrant.
3. Add the vegetable broth and chopped carrots. Bring to a boil and then reduce the heat to low and simmer for 15-20 minutes, until the carrots are tender.

4. Using an immersion blender or transferring the soup to a blender, puree the soup until smooth.
5. Stir in the salt, black pepper, Greek yogurt, and cilantro.
6. Serve hot

Nutritional information per serving (serves 4):

Calories: 140

Total fat: 5g

Saturated fat: 1g

Trans fat: 0g

Cholesterol: 3mg

Sodium: 524mg

Total carbohydrate: 19g

Dietary fiber: 5g

Sugars: 10g

Protein: 6g

Vitamin D: 0mcg

Calcium: 106mg

Iron: 2mg

Potassium: 585mg

Fennel Soup

Preparation time: 10 minutes Cooking time: 30 minutes Difficulty: Easy Portions: 4

Ingredients:
- 2 large fennel bulbs, trimmed and chopped
- 1 onion, chopped
- 2 cloves garlic, minced
- 1 tbsp olive oil
- 4 cups vegetable broth
- 1/2 cup unsweetened almond milk
- 1/2 tsp salt
- 1/4 tsp black pepper
- 1 tbsp chopped fresh parsley

Instructions:
1. Heat the olive oil in a large pot over medium heat. Add the onion and garlic and sauté for 3-4 minutes until softened.
2. Add the chopped fennel and continue to cook for an additional 5-7 minutes until the fennel is tender and slightly browned.
3. Pour in the vegetable broth and bring to a boil. Reduce the heat and simmer for 15-20 minutes until the vegetables are very tender.
4. Puree the soup with an immersion blender or transfer it to a blender and puree until smooth.
5. Return the soup to the pot and stir in the almond milk, salt, and black pepper. Heat through over low heat, stirring occasionally.
6. Serve the soup hot, garnished with chopped fresh parsley.

Nutritional Information:
- Servings: 4
- Calories per serving: 110
- Total Fat: 4.5g
- Saturated Fat: 0.6g
- Cholesterol: 0mg
- Sodium: 722mg
- Total Carbohydrates: 16.6g
- Dietary Fiber: 6.1g
- Total Sugars: 6.3g
- Protein: 3.6g

Spiced Butternut Squash Soup

Preparation Time: 15 minutes **Cooking Time:** 30 minutes **Difficulty:** Medium **Portions:** 6

Ingredients:

- 1 tablespoon olive oil
- 1 onion, chopped
- 2 garlic cloves, minced
- 1 teaspoon ground cumin
- 1 teaspoon ground coriander
- 1/2 teaspoon ground cinnamon
- 1/4 teaspoon ground nutmeg
- 1 butternut squash, peeled, seeded, and cubed (about 3 cups)
- 2 carrots, peeled and chopped
- 4 cups low-sodium vegetable broth
- 1 cup light coconut milk
- Salt and pepper to taste
- 2 tablespoons fresh cilantro, chopped
- 2 tablespoons pumpkin seeds (optional)

Instructions:

1. In a large pot or Dutch oven, heat the olive oil over medium heat. Add the chopped onion and minced garlic and sauté until the onion becomes translucent, about 5 minutes.
2. Add the ground cumin, ground coriander, ground cinnamon, and ground nutmeg to the pot. Stir well to coat the onions and garlic with the spices. Cook for an additional 1-2 minutes until fragrant.
3. Add the cubed butternut squash and chopped carrots to the pot. Stir to combine with the spices and cook for 5 minutes, allowing the vegetables to slightly soften.
4. Pour in the vegetable broth and bring the mixture to a boil. Reduce the heat to low, cover the pot, and let it simmer for about 20 minutes until the vegetables are tender.
5. Using an immersion blender or a regular blender, puree the soup until smooth and creamy. If using a regular blender, work in batches and be careful with the hot liquid.
6. Return the soup to the pot and stir in the coconut milk. Season with salt and pepper to taste. Simmer for an additional 5 minutes to heat through.
7. Serve the soup hot, garnished with chopped cilantro and pumpkin seeds (if desired).

Nutritional Information (per serving):

Calories: 160
Fat: 6g
Saturated Fat: 2g
Trans Fat: 0g
Cholesterol: 0mg
Sodium: 200mg
Carbohydrates: 26g
Fiber: 6g
Sugar: 7g
Protein: 3g
Vitamin D: 0mcg
Calcium: 84mg
Iron: 2mg
Potassium: 689mg

Roasted Tomato and Red Pepper Soup

Preparation Time: 15 minutes **Cooking Time:** 45 minutes **Difficulty:** Medium **Portions:** 4

Ingredients:

- 1 pound tomatoes, halved
- 2 red bell peppers, seeded and quartered
- 1 onion, chopped
- 3 cloves of garlic, minced
- 2 tablespoons olive oil
- 4 cups low-sodium vegetable broth
- 1 teaspoon dried basil
- 1 teaspoon dried oregano
- 1/2 teaspoon smoked paprika
- Salt and pepper to taste
- Fresh basil leaves, for garnish (optional)

Instructions:

1. Preheat the oven to 400°F (200°C).
2. Place the halved tomatoes and quartered red bell peppers on a baking sheet. Drizzle with olive oil and sprinkle with salt and pepper. Roast in the preheated oven for 25-30 minutes until the vegetables are softened and slightly charred.
3. In a large pot or Dutch oven, heat the remaining olive oil over medium heat. Add the chopped onion and minced garlic. Sauté until the onion becomes translucent, about 5 minutes.
4. Add the roasted tomatoes and red bell peppers to the pot, along with any juices from the baking sheet. Stir in the dried basil, dried oregano, smoked paprika, salt, and pepper.
5. Pour in the vegetable broth and bring the mixture to a boil. Reduce the heat to low, cover the pot, and let it simmer for 15 minutes to allow the flavors to meld together
6. Using an immersion blender or a regular blender, puree the soup until smooth and creamy. If using a regular blender, work in batches and be careful with the hot liquid.
7. Return the soup to the pot and simmer for an additional 5 minutes to heat through.
8. Serve the soup hot, garnished with fresh basil leaves if desired.

Nutritional Information (per serving):

Calories: 130
Fat: 7g
Saturated Fat: 1g
Trans Fat: 0g
Cholesterol: 0mg
Sodium: 283mg
Carbohydrates: 16g
Fiber: 4g
Sugar: 9g
Protein: 3g
Vitamin D: 0mcg
Calcium: 32mg
Iron: 1mg
Potassium: 550mg

SIDES RECIPES

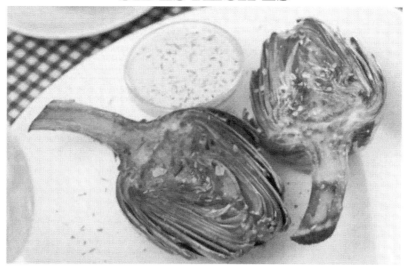

Roasted Balsamic Brussels Sprouts with Cranberries

Preparation Time: 10 minutes **Cooking Time:** 25 minutes **Difficulty:** Easy **Servings:** 4

Ingredients:

- 1 pound Brussels sprouts, trimmed and halved
- 1/2 cup dried cranberries
- 2 tablespoons balsamic vinegar
- 2 tablespoons olive oil
- 1 tablespoon honey
- 1/2 teaspoon salt
- 1/4 teaspoon black pepper
- 1/4 cup chopped pecans (optional)

Instructions:

1. Preheat the oven to 400°F (200°C).
2. In a large bowl, combine the balsamic vinegar, olive oil, honey, salt, and black pepper. Whisk together until well combined.
3. Add the halved Brussels sprouts and dried cranberries to the bowl. Toss to coat them evenly with the balsamic mixture.
4. Transfer the Brussels sprouts and cranberries to a baking sheet, spreading them out in a single layer.
5. Roast in the preheated oven for 20-25 minutes, or until the Brussels sprouts are tender and slightly caramelized, stirring once halfway through.
6. Optional: In a small pan over medium heat, toast the chopped pecans for a few minutes until fragrant.
7. Remove the roasted Brussels sprouts from the oven and transfer them to a serving dish. Sprinkle with the toasted pecans (if using).
8. Serve the roasted Brussels sprouts as a delicious and unique side dish.

Nutritional Information (per serving):

Calories: 178

Fat: 8g

Saturated Fat: 1g

Trans Fat: 0g

Cholesterol: 0mg

Sodium: 309mg

Carbohydrates: 26g

Fiber: 6g

Sugar: 14g

Protein: 4g

Lemon Garlic Roasted Asparagus

Preparation Time: 10 minutes **Cooking Time:** 15 minutes **Difficulty:** Easy **Servings:** 4

Ingredients:

- 1 pound asparagus spears, trimmed
- 2 tablespoons olive oil
- 2 cloves garlic, minced
- Zest of 1 lemon
- 1 tablespoon lemon juice
- 1/2 teaspoon salt
- 1/4 teaspoon black pepper
- Lemon wedges, for garnish (optional)

Instructions:

1. Preheat the oven to 425°F (220°C).
2. In a small bowl, combine the olive oil, minced garlic, lemon zest, lemon juice, salt, and black pepper. Mix well.
3. Place the trimmed asparagus spears on a baking sheet lined with parchment paper.
4. Drizzle the asparagus with the lemon garlic mixture, tossing to ensure all the spears are coated evenly.
5. Spread the asparagus out in a single layer on the baking sheet.
6. Roast in the preheated oven for about 12-15 minutes, or until the asparagus is tender and slightly charred, stirring once halfway through.
7. Remove from the oven and transfer the roasted asparagus to a serving dish.
8. Garnish with lemon wedges, if desired, and serve hot as a delightful side dish.

Nutritional Information (per serving):

Calories: 82

Fat: 7g

Saturated Fat: 1g

Trans Fat: 0g

Cholesterol: 0mg

Sodium: 295mg

Carbohydrates: 5g

Fiber: 3g

Sugar: 2g

Protein: 3g

Balsamic Roasted Green Beans with Parmesan

Preparation Time: 10 minutes **Cooking Time:** 20 minutes **Difficulty:** Easy **Servings:** 4

Ingredients:

- 1 pound green beans, trimmed
- 2 tablespoons balsamic vinegar
- 2 tablespoons olive oil
- 2 cloves garlic, minced
- 1/2 teaspoon salt
- 1/4 teaspoon black pepper
- 1/4 cup grated Parmesan cheese

Instructions:

1. Preheat the oven to 425°F (220°C).
2. In a small bowl, whisk together the balsamic vinegar, olive oil, minced garlic, salt, and black pepper.
3. Place the trimmed green beans on a baking sheet lined with parchment paper.
4. Drizzle the balsamic mixture over the green beans, tossing to coat them evenly
5. Spread the green beans out in a single layer on the baking sheet.
6. Roast in the preheated oven for about 15-20 minutes, or until the green beans are tender and slightly caramelized, stirring once halfway through.
7. Remove from the oven and sprinkle the grated Parmesan cheese over the roasted green beans. Toss gently to combine.
8. Serve the balsamic roasted green beans with Parmesan as a delightful and flavorful side dish.

Nutritional Information (per serving):

Calories: 108

Fat: 7g

Saturated Fat: 2g

Trans Fat: 0g

Cholesterol: 6mg

Sodium: 369mg

Carbohydrates: 8g

Fiber: 3g

Sugar: 4g

Protein: 4g

Garlic Herb Mashed Potatoes

Preparation Time: 15 minutes **Cooking Time**: 20 minutes **Difficulty**: Easy **Servings**: 4

Ingredients:

- 2 pounds potatoes (such as Russet or Yukon Gold), peeled and cut into chunks
- 4 cloves garlic, minced
- 1/2 cup milk (or dairy-free alternative)
- 4 tablespoons unsalted butter (or dairy-free alternative)
- 2 tablespoons fresh parsley, chopped
- 1 tablespoon fresh chives, chopped
- 1/2 teaspoon dried thyme
- Salt and pepper, to taste

Instructions:

1. Place the potato chunks in a large pot and cover with cold water. Add a pinch of salt to the water. Bring to a boil over high heat and cook until the potatoes are fork-tender, about 15-20 minutes.
2. While the potatoes are cooking, melt the butter in a small saucepan over low heat. Add the minced garlic and sauté for 1-2 minutes until fragrant. Set aside.
3. Drain the cooked potatoes and return them to the pot. Add the garlic butter mixture, milk, parsley, chives, dried thyme, salt, and pepper.
4. Using a potato masher or an electric mixer, mash the potatoes until smooth and creamy. Adjust the consistency by adding more milk if needed. Taste and adjust the seasoning with salt and pepper.
5. Transfer the mashed potatoes to a serving dish.
6. Serve the garlic herb mashed potatoes hot as a delectable side dish alongside your favorite main course.

Nutritional Information (per serving):

Calories: 252
Fat: 11g
Saturated Fat: 7g
Trans Fat: 0g
Cholesterol: 30mg
Sodium: 43mg
Carbohydrates: 34g
Fiber: 4g
Sugar: 2g
Protein: 4g

Fennel and Orange Salad

Preparation Time: 10 minutes **Difficulty**: Easy **Servings:** 4

Ingredients:

- 2 large fennel bulbs
- 2 oranges
- 1/4 cup extra-virgin olive oil
- 2 tablespoons fresh lemon juice
- 1 teaspoon Dijon mustard
- Salt and pepper, to taste
- Fresh mint leaves, for garnish (optional)

Instructions:

1. Trim the fronds off the fennel bulbs and remove any tough outer layers. Cut the bulbs in half lengthwise, then thinly slice them crosswise.
2. Peel the oranges, removing the pith, and cut them into segments.
3. In a small bowl, whisk together the olive oil, lemon juice, Dijon mustard, salt, and pepper to make the dressing.
4. In a large salad bowl, combine the sliced fennel and orange segments.
5. Drizzle the dressing over the fennel and oranges. Toss gently to coat.
6. Let the salad sit for a few minutes to allow the flavors to meld together.
7. Garnish with fresh mint leaves, if desired.
8. Serve the fennel and orange salad as a refreshing and vibrant side dish.

Fennel and Orange Salad

Preparation Time: 10 minutes **Difficulty**: Easy **Servings:** 4

Ingredients:

- 2 large fennel bulbs
- 2 oranges
- 1/4 cup extra-virgin olive oil
- 2 tablespoons fresh lemon juice
- 1 teaspoon Dijon mustard
- Salt and pepper, to taste
- Fresh mint leaves, for garnish (optional)

Nutritional Information (per serving):

Calories: 121

Fat: 10g

Saturated Fat: 1g

Trans Fat: 0g

Cholesterol: 0mg

Sodium: 40mg

Carbohydrates: 9g

Fiber: 4g

Sugar: 4g

Protein: 1g

Ratatouille

Preparation Time: 15 minutes **Cooking Time:** 40 minutes **Difficulty:** Easy **Servings:** 4

Ingredients:

- 1 medium eggplant, cut into 1-inch cubes
- 2 medium zucchini, sliced
- 1 red bell pepper, sliced
- 1 yellow bell pepper, sliced
- 1 onion, sliced
- 3 cloves garlic, minced
- 3 tablespoons olive oil
- 1 can (14 ounces) diced tomatoes
- 1 teaspoon dried basil
- 1 teaspoon dried thyme
- 1/2 teaspoon dried oregano
- Salt and pepper, to taste
- Fresh basil leaves, for garnish (optional)

Instructions:

1. Preheat the oven to 375°F (190°C).
2. In a large baking dish, combine the eggplant, zucchini, bell peppers, onion, and minced garlic.
3. Drizzle the vegetables with olive oil and season with salt and pepper. Toss to coat the vegetables evenly.
4. Bake in the preheated oven for about 20 minutes, or until the vegetables start to soften.
5. Remove the baking dish from the oven and add the diced tomatoes, dried basil, dried thyme, dried oregano, and additional salt and pepper to taste. Gently stir to combine.
6. Return the baking dish to the oven and continue baking for another 15-20 minutes, or until the vegetables are tender and slightly caramelized.
7. Remove from the oven and let the ratatouille cool slightly.
8. Garnish with fresh basil leaves, if desired, and serve the ratatouille as a flavorful and hearty side dish.

Nutritional Information (per serving):

Calories: 164
Fat: 10g
Saturated Fat: 1g
Trans Fat: 0g
Cholesterol: 0mg
Sodium: 412mg

Carbohydrates: 18g
Fiber: 6g
Sugar: 9g
Protein: 3g

Courgette Pizza

Preparation Time: 15 minutes **Cooking Time:** 25 minutes **Difficulty:** Easy **Servings:** 4

Ingredients:

- 2 large courgettes (zucchini), sliced into 1/4-inch rounds
- 1/4 cup pizza sauce or marinara sauce
- 1/2 cup shredded mozzarella cheese
- 1/4 cup sliced cherry tomatoes
- 1/4 cup sliced black olives
- 1/4 cup sliced mushrooms
- Fresh basil leaves, for garnish
- Olive oil, for drizzling
- Salt and pepper, to taste

Instructions:

1. Preheat the oven to 425°F (220°C).
2. Place the courgette rounds on a baking sheet lined with parchment paper. Drizzle with olive oil and season with salt and pepper.
3. Bake the courgette rounds in the preheated oven for about 10 minutes, or until slightly softened.
4. Remove the courgette rounds from the oven and spread a thin layer of pizza sauce or marinara sauce on each round.
5. Sprinkle shredded mozzarella cheese over the sauce.
6. Top with sliced cherry tomatoes, black olives, and sliced mushrooms, or any other desired pizza toppings.
7. Return the baking sheet to the oven and bake for another 10-15 minutes, or until the cheese is melted and bubbly.
8. Remove from the oven and garnish with fresh basil leaves.
9. Serve the courgette pizza slices hot as a delicious and low-carb side dish or appetizer.

Nutritional Information (per serving):

Calories: 109
Fat: 7g
Saturated Fat: 2g
Trans Fat: 0g
Cholesterol: 10mg

Sodium: 299mg
Carbohydrates: 6g
Fiber: 2g
Sugar: 4g
Protein: 6g

Baked Peppers with Capers

Preparation Time: 10 minutes **Cooking Time:** 25 minutes **Difficulty:** Easy **Servings:** 4

Ingredients:

- 4 bell peppers (any color), halved and seeds removed
- 2 tablespoons capers, drained
- 2 cloves garlic, minced
- 2 tablespoons olive oil
- 1 tablespoon balsamic vinegar
- 1 teaspoon dried oregano
- Salt and pepper, to taste
- Fresh parsley, for garnish

Instructions:

1. Preheat the oven to 400°F (200°C).
2. Place the bell pepper halves on a baking sheet lined with parchment paper.
3. In a small bowl, mix together the capers, minced garlic, olive oil, balsamic vinegar, dried oregano, salt, and pepper.
4. Spoon the caper mixture evenly into each bell pepper half.
5. Place the baking sheet in the preheated oven and bake for about 20-25 minutes, or until the peppers are tender and slightly charred.
6. Remove from the oven and let the baked peppers cool slightly.
7. Garnish with fresh parsley.
8. Serve the baked peppers with capers as a delicious and tangy side dish that pairs well with grilled meats or as a topping for salads.

Nutritional Information (per serving):

Calories: 101
Fat: 7g
Saturated Fat: 1g
Trans Fat: 0g
Cholesterol: 0mg

Sodium: 249mg
Carbohydrates: 10g
Fiber: 3g
Sugar: 6g
Protein: 2g

Grilled Artichokes with Lemon Garlic Dip

Preparation Time: 15 minutes **Cooking Time:** 25 minutes **Difficulty:** Easy **Servings:** 4

Ingredients:

- 4 large artichokes
- 1 lemon, halved
- 4 tablespoons olive oil
- Salt and pepper, to taste

For the Lemon Garlic Dip:

- 1/2 cup mayonnaise
- 1 clove garlic, minced
- 1 tablespoon fresh lemon juice
- 1 teaspoon lemon zest
- Salt and pepper, to taste
- Salt and pepper, to taste

Instructions:

1. Fill a large pot with water and squeeze the juice from one lemon half into the water. Bring the water to a boil.
2. Trim the stems of the artichokes and remove any tough outer leaves. Cut off the top third of each artichoke and use kitchen shears to trim the sharp tips of the remaining leaves.
3. Place the artichokes in the boiling water and cook for about 15-20 minutes, or until the base is tender when pierced with a fork. Drain and set aside.
4. Preheat the grill to medium-high heat.
5. In a small bowl, combine the olive oil, juice from the remaining lemon half, salt, and pepper. Brush the mixture onto the artichokes, making sure to coat all sides.

6. Place the artichokes on the grill and cook for about 5-7 minutes per side, or until they develop grill marks and become tender.
7. While the artichokes are grilling, prepare the Lemon Garlic Dip. In a bowl, combine the mayonnaise, minced garlic, lemon juice, lemon zest, salt, and pepper. Stir until well combined.
8. Remove the grilled artichokes from the grill and serve them hot with the Lemon Garlic Dip on the side.

Nutritional Information (per serving):

Calories: 253

Fat: 22g

Saturated Fat: 3g

Trans Fat: 0g

Cholesterol: 8mg

Sodium: 307mg

Carbohydrates: 13g

Fiber: 6g

Sugar: 1g

Protein: 2g

Stewed Peas with Bacon

Preparation Time: 10 minutes **Cooking Time:** 25 minutes **Difficulty:** Easy **Servings:** 4

Ingredients:

- 4 slices bacon, chopped
- 1 small onion, diced
- 2 cloves garlic, minced
- 2 cups frozen peas

- 1 cup chicken or vegetable broth
- 1 teaspoon dried thyme
- Salt and pepper, to taste
- Fresh parsley, for garnish (optional)

Instructions:

1. In a large skillet or pan, cook the chopped bacon over medium heat until crispy. Remove the bacon from the pan and set it aside on a paper towel-lined plate to drain.
2. In the same pan with the bacon drippings, add the diced onion and minced garlic. Sauté until the onion becomes translucent and fragrant, about 3-4 minutes.
3. Add the frozen peas to the pan and stir them in with the onion and garlic.
4. Pour in the chicken or vegetable broth and add the dried thyme. Season with salt and pepper to taste.
5. Bring the mixture to a simmer and let it cook for about 15-20 minutes, or until the peas are tender and the flavors have melded together.
6. Once the peas are cooked to your desired tenderness, remove the pan from heat.
7. Stir in the cooked bacon, reserving a small amount for garnish if desired.
8. Serve the stewed peas with bacon hot, garnished with fresh parsley if desired.

Nutritional Information (per serving):

Calories: 126

Fat: 6g

Saturated Fat: 2g

Trans Fat: 0g

Cholesterol: 10mg

Sodium: 415mg

Carbohydrates: 11g

Fiber: 3g

Sugar: 4g

Protein: 7g

SALAD RECIPES
Greek Salad

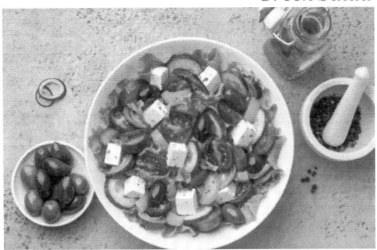

Preparation Time: 15 minutes **Difficulty**: Easy **Servings:** 4

Ingredients:

- 2 large tomatoes, cut into chunks
- 1 cucumber, sliced
- 1 red onion, thinly sliced
- 1 green bell pepper, sliced
- 1/2 cup Kalamata olives, pitted
- 1/2 cup crumbled vegan feta cheese (optional)
- 1/4 cup extra virgin olive oil
- 2 tablespoons red wine vinegar
- 1 teaspoon dried oregano
- Salt and pepper, to taste
- Fresh parsley, chopped (for garnish)

Instructions:

1. In a large salad bowl, combine the tomato chunks, sliced cucumber, thinly sliced red onion, and sliced green bell pepper.
2. Add the Kalamata olives to the bowl. If desired, crumble the vegan feta cheese over the salad.
3. In a small bowl, whisk together the extra virgin olive oil, red wine vinegar, dried oregano, salt, and pepper. Adjust the seasonings to taste.
4. Pour the dressing over the salad and toss gently to coat all the ingredients.
5. Let the Greek salad sit for a few minutes to allow the flavors to meld together.
6. Garnish with fresh chopped parsley.
7. Serve the Greek salad as a refreshing and nutritious side dish or as a light main course.

Nutritional Information (per serving)

Calories: 162

Fat: 13g

Saturated Fat: 2g

Trans Fat: 0g

Cholesterol: 0mg

Sodium: 329mg

Carbohydrates: 10g

Fiber: 3g

Sugar: 5g

Protein: 2g

Aeolian salad Sicilian style

Preparation Time: 15 minutes **Difficulty**: Easy **Servings**: 4

Ingredients:

- 2 cups cherry tomatoes, halved
- 1 English cucumber, diced
- 1 red bell pepper, diced
- 1/2 red onion, thinly sliced
- 1/2 cup Kalamata olives, pitted and halved
- 1/4 cup fresh basil leaves, torn
- Vegan feta cheese, crumbled (optional)
- 1/4 cup fresh mint leaves, torn
- 1/4 cup extra virgin olive oil
- 2 tablespoons red wine vinegar
- 1 teaspoon dried oregano
- Salt and pepper, to taste

Instructions:

1. In a large salad bowl, combine the cherry tomatoes, diced cucumber, diced red bell pepper, thinly sliced red onion, and halved Kalamata olives.
2. Add the torn fresh basil leaves and fresh mint leaves to the bowl.
3. In a small bowl, whisk together the extra virgin olive oil, red wine vinegar, dried oregano, salt, and pepper. Adjust the seasonings to taste.
4. Pour the dressing over the salad and toss gently to coat all the ingredients.
5. Let the Aeolian salad sit for a few minutes to allow the flavors to meld together.
6. If desired, crumble some vegan feta cheese over the salad for added flavor.

Nutritional Information (per serving):

Calories: 157
Fat: 12g
Saturated Fat: 2g
Trans Fat: 0g
Cholesterol: 0mg

Sodium: 232mg
Carbohydrates: 12g
Fiber: 3g
Sugar: 6g
Protein: 2g

Melon Salad

Preparation Time: 15 minutes **Difficulty**: Easy **Servings**: 4

Ingredients:

- 4 cups cubed melon (watermelon, honeydew, or cantaloupe, or a mix)
- 1 cup fresh berries (strawberries, blueberries, or raspberries)
- 1/4 cup fresh mint leaves, chopped
- 1 tablespoon fresh lime juice
- 1 tablespoon honey (or maple syrup for a vegan option)
- 1/4 cup chopped pistachios (optional, for garnish)
- Fresh mint leaves (for garnish)

Instructions:

1. In a large bowl, combine the cubed melon and fresh berries.
2. In a small bowl, whisk together the fresh lime juice and honey (or maple syrup) to create the dressing.
3. Pour the dressing over the melon and berries, and gently toss to coat
4. Add the chopped mint leaves to the bowl and gently toss again to distribute the flavors.
5. Garnish the melon salad with chopped pistachios (if using) and additional fresh mint leaves.

Nutritional Information (per serving):

Calories: 84
Fat: 1g
Saturated Fat: 0g
Trans Fat: 0g
Cholesterol: 0mg

Sodium: 9mg
Carbohydrates: 21g
Fiber: 2g
Sugar: 18g
Protein: 1g

Salmon, Orange, and Fennel Salad

Preparation Time: 20 minutes **Cooking Time**: 10 minutes **Difficulty**: Easy **Servings**: 4

Ingredients:

- 4 salmon fillets (about 4-6 ounces each)
- Salt and pepper, to taste
- 2 tablespoons olive oil
- 1 large fennel bulb, thinly sliced
- 2 oranges, peeled and segmented
- 4 cups mixed salad greens
- 1/4 cup sliced almonds, toasted

- For the dressing:
- 2 tablespoons orange juice
- 1 tablespoon lemon juice
- 2 tablespoons extra virgin olive oil
- 1 teaspoon Dijon mustard
- Salt and pepper, to taste

Instructions:

Preheat the oven to 400°F (200°C). Season the salmon fillets with salt and pepper.

Heat the olive oil in an oven-safe skillet over medium-high heat. Place the salmon fillets in the skillet, skin-side down, and cook for about 3-4 minutes until the skin is crispy.

Transfer the skillet to the preheated oven and bake for an additional 5-6 minutes, or until the salmon is cooked through and flakes easily with a fork. Remove from the oven and set aside to cool slightly.

In a large bowl, combine the sliced fennel, orange segments, and mixed salad greens.

In a small bowl, whisk together the orange juice, lemon juice, extra virgin olive oil, Dijon mustard, salt, and pepper to make the dressing.

Pour the dressing over the salad ingredients and toss gently to coat.

Divide the salad among serving plates and top each plate with a salmon fillet.

Sprinkle with toasted sliced almonds for added crunch and flavor.

Nutritional Information (per serving):

- Calories: 355
- Fat: 23g
- Saturated Fat: 3g
- Trans Fat: 0g
- Cholesterol: 50mg

- Sodium: 134mg
- Carbohydrates: 16g
- Fiber: 6g
- Sugar: 8g
- Protein: 23g

Chickpea and Shrimp Salad

Preparation Time: 15 minutes **Cooking Time**: 5 minutes **Difficulty**: Easy **Servings**: 4

Ingredients:

- 1 pound shrimp, peeled and deveined
- 2 tablespoons olive oil
- Salt and pepper, to taste
- 1 can chickpeas (15 ounces), drained and rinsed
- 1 cup cherry tomatoes, halved
- 1 cucumber, diced
- 1/4 cup red onion, finely chopped

- 1/4 cup fresh parsley, chopped
- Juice of 1 lemon
- 2 tablespoons extra virgin olive oil
- 1 teaspoon Dijon mustard
- 1 clove garlic, minced
- Salt and pepper, to taste
- Mixed salad greens (optional, for serving)

Instructions:

1. In a large skillet, heat the olive oil over medium-high heat. Season the shrimp with salt and pepper, then add them to the skillet. Cook the shrimp for about 2-3 minutes per side until pink and cooked through. Remove from heat and set aside to cool
2. In a large bowl, combine the chickpeas, cherry tomatoes, diced cucumber, red onion, and fresh parsley.
3. In a small bowl, whisk together the lemon juice, extra virgin olive oil, Dijon mustard, minced garlic, salt, and pepper to make the dressing.
4. Pour the dressing over the chickpea and vegetable mixture. Toss gently to coat all the ingredients.
5. Add the cooked shrimp to the bowl and gently toss to incorporate.
6. If desired, serve the chickpea and shrimp salad on a bed of mixed salad greens for added freshness and presentation.

Nutritional Information (per serving):

Calories: 281

Fat: 11g

Saturated Fat: 2g

Trans Fat: 0g

Cholesterol: 191mg

Sodium: 652mg

Carbohydrates: 22g

Fiber: 5g

Sugar: 4g

Protein: 26g

Potato, Carrot, and Rocket Pesto Salad

Preparation Time: 15 minutes **Cooking Time:** 20 minutes **Difficulty:** Easy **Servings:** 4

Ingredients:

- 4 medium potatoes, peeled and cubed
- 2 carrots, peeled and sliced
- 2 cups rocket (arugula) leaves
- 1/4 cup pine nuts, toasted
- 2 cloves garlic, minced
- 1/4 cup extra virgin olive oil
- Juice of 1 lemon
- Salt and pepper, to taste

Instructions:

1. In a large pot, bring water to a boil. Add the cubed potatoes and sliced carrots, and cook until tender, about 10-12 minutes. Drain and set aside to cool.
2. In a food processor, combine the rocket leaves, toasted pine nuts, minced garlic, extra virgin olive oil, lemon juice, salt, and pepper. Blend until a smooth pesto-like consistency is achieved.
3. In a large mixing bowl, combine the cooked and cooled potatoes and carrots. Add the rocket pesto and toss gently to coat the vegetables evenly.
4. Taste and adjust the seasoning if needed. You can add more lemon juice, salt, or pepper according to your preference.

Nutritional Information (per serving):

Calories: 258

Fat: 15g

Saturated Fat: 2g

Trans Fat: 0g

Cholesterol: 0mg

Sodium: 33mg

Carbohydrates: 28g

Fiber: 4g

Sugar: 2g

Protein: 4g

Tuna Fish Salad

Preparation Time: 10 minutes **Difficulty:** Easy **Servings:** 4

Ingredients:

- 2 cans (5 ounces each) tuna in water, drained
- 1/4 cup mayonnaise
- 2 tablespoons plain Greek yogurt (or sour cream)
- 1 tablespoon lemon juice
- 1/4 cup finely chopped celery
- 2 tablespoons finely chopped red onion
- 2 tablespoons chopped fresh parsley
- Salt and pepper, to taste
- Lettuce leaves (for serving)
- Sliced tomatoes (for serving)
- Sliced cucumbers (for serving)

Instructions:

In a medium bowl, flake the drained tuna using a fork.

Add the mayonnaise, Greek yogurt (or sour cream), lemon juice, chopped celery, chopped red onion, and chopped parsley to the bowl with the tuna. Mix well to combine all the ingredients.

Season the tuna salad with salt and pepper to taste. Adjust the amount of mayo or Greek yogurt based on your preferred creaminess.

Place lettuce leaves on a serving plate or individual plates. Top with the tuna salad.

Nutritional Information (per serving):

- Calories: 214
- Fat: 12g
- Saturated Fat: 2g
- Trans Fat: 0g
- Cholesterol: 39mg
- Sodium: 386mg
- Carbohydrates: 3g
- Fiber: 1g
- Sugar: 1g
- Protein: 23g

BREAD RECIPES
Whole Wheat Bread

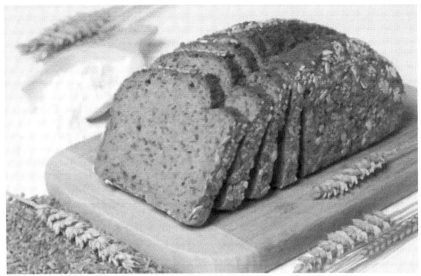

Preparation Time: 2 hours 30 minutes **Cooking Time:** 40 minutes **Difficulty:** Moderate **Servings:** 12 slices

Ingredients:

- 2 cups whole wheat flour
- 1 cup all-purpose flour
- 1 packet (2 1/4 teaspoons) active dry yeast
- 1 teaspoon salt
- 1 tablespoon honey
- 1 1/4 cups warm water (110°F/43°C)
- Cooking spray (for greasing)

Instructions:

1. In a large mixing bowl, combine the whole wheat flour, all-purpose flour, yeast, and salt.
2. In a separate bowl, mix together the honey and warm water until the honey is dissolved.
3. Add the honey-water mixture to the flour mixture and stir until a dough forms.
4. Turn the dough out onto a floured surface and knead for about 5-7 minutes until smooth and elastic.
5. Place the dough in a greased bowl, cover with a clean kitchen towel, and let it rise in a warm place for about 1-1.5 hours until doubled in size.
6. Preheat the oven to 375°F (190°C). Punch down the dough and shape it into a loaf.
7. Place the loaf in a greased loaf pan, cover again with the towel, and let it rise for an additional 30 minutes.
8. Bake the bread for about 35-40 minutes until golden brown and sounds hollow when tapped on the bottom.
9. Remove the bread from the pan and let it cool completely on a wire rack before slicing.

Nutritional Information (per slice):

Calories: 128
Fat: 0.7g
Saturated Fat: 0.1g
Trans Fat: 0g
Cholesterol: 0mg
Sodium: 195mg
Carbohydrates: 27.3g
Fiber: 3.9g
Sugar: 1.2g
Protein: 4.7g

Oatmeal Bread

Preparation Time: 2 hours 30 minutes **Cooking Time**: 40 minutes **Difficulty**: Moderate **Servings**: 12 slices

Ingredients:

- 1 1/2 cups old-fashioned rolled oats
- 1 1/2 cups boiling water
- 2 tablespoons honey
- 2 tablespoons olive oil
- 2 teaspoons active dry yeast
- 1 1/2 cups whole wheat flour
- 1 1/2 cups all-purpose flour
- 1 teaspoon salt

Instructions:

1. In a large bowl, combine the rolled oats, boiling water, honey, and olive oil. Stir well and let it sit for about 20 minutes until the mixture cools down.
2. Sprinkle the yeast over the oat mixture and let it sit for 5 minutes until it becomes frothy.
3. Add the whole wheat flour, all-purpose flour, and salt to the bowl. Stir until the dough comes together.
4. Transfer the dough onto a lightly floured surface and knead for about 5-7 minutes until it becomes smooth and elastic. Add more flour if needed to prevent sticking.
5. Shape the dough into a ball and place it in a greased bowl. Cover with a clean kitchen towel and let it rise in a warm place for about 1-1.5 hours until it doubles in size.
6. Preheat the oven to 400°F (200°C). Grease a loaf pan with olive oil or cooking spray.
7. Punch down the dough to release any air bubbles and transfer it to the greased loaf pan. Press the dough down evenly into the pan.
8. Cover the pan with the kitchen towel and let it rise for another 30 minutes.
9. Bake the bread in the preheated oven for 35-40 minutes or until it turns golden brown and sounds hollow when tapped on the bottom.
10. Remove the bread from the oven and let it cool in the pan for a few minutes. Then transfer it to a wire rack to cool completely before slicing.
11. Enjoy the homemade oatmeal bread as a nutritious and hearty addition to your DASH diet.

Nutritional Information (per slice):

Calories: 146
Fat: 3.6g
Saturated Fat: 0.5g
Trans Fat: 0g
Cholesterol: 0mg

Sodium: 196mg
Carbohydrates: 26.7g
Fiber: 3.6g
Sugar: 2.3g
Protein: 4.7g

Quinoa Bread

Preparation Time: 15 minutes **Cooking Time:** 1 hour **Difficulty:** Moderate **Servings:** 12 slices

Ingredients:

- 1 1/2 cups cooked quinoa, cooled
- 1 1/2 cups whole wheat flour
- 1/2 cup oat flour
- 1/4 cup ground flaxseed
- 2 teaspoons baking powder
- 1/2 teaspoon salt
- 1/2 teaspoon dried herbs (such as thyme or rosemary)
- 1 cup unsweetened almond milk (or any plant-based milk)
- 2 tablespoons maple syrup
- 2 tablespoons olive oil
- 1 tablespoon apple cider vinegar

Instructions:

1. Preheat the oven to 350°F (175°C). Grease a 9x5-inch loaf pan with cooking spray.
2. In a large bowl, whisk together the whole wheat flour, oat flour, ground flaxseed, baking powder, salt, and dried herbs.
3. In a separate bowl, mix together the cooked quinoa, almond milk, maple syrup, olive oil, and apple cider vinegar.
4. Pour the wet ingredients into the dry ingredients and stir until well combined.
5. Transfer the batter to the greased loaf pan and smooth the top.
6. Bake for about 50-60 minutes, or until a toothpick inserted into the center comes out clean.

7. Remove the bread from the oven and let it cool in the pan for about 10 minutes. Then, transfer the bread to a wire rack to cool completely before slicing.

Nutritional Information (per slice):

Calories: 144
Fat: 3.9g
Saturated Fat: 0.5g
Trans Fat: 0g
Cholesterol: 0mg
Sodium: 198mg

Carbohydrates: 23.5g
Fiber: 4.2g
Sugar: 2.6g
Protein: 4.6g

Cereal Bread

Preparation Time: 2 hours 30 minutes **Cooking Time:** 40 minutes **Difficulty:** Moderate **Servings:** 12 slices

Ingredients:

- 1 cup whole wheat flour
- 1 cup all-purpose flour
- 1 cup whole grain cereal (such as wheat flakes or rolled oats)
- 1/4 cup ground flaxseed
- 2 teaspoons active dry yeast
- 1 teaspoon salt
- 1 tablespoon honey
- 1 cup warm water (110°F/43°C)
- 2 tablespoons olive oil
- Cooking spray (for greasing)

Instructions:

1. In a large mixing bowl, combine the whole wheat flour, all-purpose flour, whole grain cereal, ground flaxseed, yeast, and salt.
2. In a separate bowl, mix together the honey and warm water until the honey is dissolved. Add the olive oil and stir to combine.
3. Pour the liquid mixture into the dry ingredients and stir until a dough forms. If the dough is too sticky, add a little more flour.
4. Transfer the dough to a lightly floured surface and knead for about 5-7 minutes until smooth and elastic.
5. Place the dough in a greased bowl, cover with a clean kitchen towel, and let it rise in a warm place for about 1-1.5 hours until doubled in size.
6. Preheat the oven to 375°F (190°C). Punch down the dough and shape it into a loaf.
7. Place the loaf in a greased loaf pan, cover again with the towel, and let it rise for an additional 30 minutes.
8. Bake the bread for about 35-40 minutes until golden brown and sounds hollow when tapped on the bottom.
9. Remove the bread from the pan and let it cool completely on a wire rack before slicing.

Nutritional Information (per slice):

Calories: 132
Fat: 3.5g
Saturated Fat: 0.5g
Trans Fat: 0g
Cholesterol: 0mg
Sodium: 196mg
Carbohydrates: 22.4g
Fiber: 3.6g
Sugar: 2g
Protein: 4.2g

Rye and Seed Bread

Preparation Time: 2 hours 30 minutes **Cooking Time:** 40 minutes **Difficulty:** Moderate **Servings:** 12 slices

Ingredients:

- 2 cups rye flour
- 1 1/2 cups whole wheat flour
- 1/2 cup sunflower seeds
- 1/4 cup pumpkin seeds
- 2 tablespoons flaxseeds
- 2 teaspoons caraway seeds
- 2 teaspoons active dry yeast
- 1 teaspoon salt
- 1 tablespoon honey or maple syrup
- 1 1/4 cups warm water (110°F/43°C)
- 2 tablespoons olive oil
- Cooking spray (for greasing)

Instructions:

1. In a large mixing bowl, combine the rye flour, whole wheat flour, sunflower seeds, pumpkin seeds, flaxseeds, caraway seeds, yeast, and salt.
2. In a separate bowl, dissolve the honey or maple syrup in warm water. Add the olive oil and stir to combine.
3. Pour the liquid mixture into the dry ingredients and stir until a dough forms. If the dough is too sticky, add a little more flour.
4. Transfer the dough to a lightly floured surface and knead for about 5-7 minutes until smooth and elastic.
5. Place the dough in a greased bowl, cover with a clean kitchen towel, and let it rise in a warm place for about 1-1.5 hours until doubled in size.
6. Preheat the oven to 375°F (190°C). Punch down the dough and shape it into a loaf.
7. Place the loaf in a greased loaf pan, cover again with the towel, and let it rise for an additional 30 minutes.
8. Bake the bread for about 35-40 minutes until golden brown and sounds hollow when tapped on the bottom.
9. Remove the bread from the pan and let it cool completely on a wire rack before slicing.

Nutritional Information (per slice):

Calories: 154
Fat: 6.4g
Saturated Fat: 0.8g
Trans Fat: 0g
Cholesterol: 0mg

Sodium: 200mg
Carbohydrates: 21.3
Fiber: 4.3g
Sugar: 1.8g
Protein: 5.5g

SNACKS & APPETIZER RECIPES
Peanut Butter Energy Bars

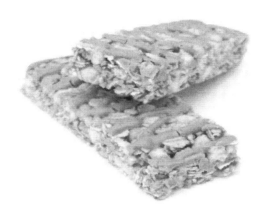

Preparation Time: 10 minutes **Chilling Time:** 1 hour **Difficulty:** Easy **Servings:** 12 bars

Ingredients:

- 1 1/2 cups old-fashioned rolled oats
- 1/2 cup natural peanut butter
- 1/3 cup honey or maple syrup
- 1/4 cup unsweetened shredded coconut
- 1/4 cup chopped nuts (e.g., almonds, walnuts)
- 1/4 cup dried cranberries or raisins
- 1/4 cup mini chocolate chips (optional)
- 1 teaspoon vanilla extract
- Pinch of salt

Instructions:

1. In a large mixing bowl, combine the rolled oats, peanut butter, honey or maple syrup, shredded coconut, chopped nuts, dried cranberries or raisins, mini chocolate chips (if using), vanilla extract, and salt. Stir well until all the ingredients are evenly mixed.
2. Line an 8x8-inch baking dish with parchment paper or lightly grease it with cooking spray.
3. Transfer the mixture into the prepared baking dish. Use a spatula or your hands to press the mixture firmly and evenly into the dish.
4. Place the dish in the refrigerator and chill for at least 1 hour to firm up.
5. Once chilled, remove the mixture from the dish and cut it into 12 bars.
6. Individually wrap the bars in plastic wrap or store them in an airtight container in the refrigerator for up to 2 weeks.

Nutritional Information (per bar):

Calories: 186

Fat: 9.7g

Saturated Fat: 2.1g

Trans Fat: 0g

Cholesterol: 0mg

Sodium: 41mg

Carbohydrates: 22g

Fiber: 2.8g

Sugar: 11.7g

Protein: 5.3g

Vitamin D: 0mcg

Calcium: 16mg

Iron: 1mg

Potassium: 184mg

No-Bake Almond Date Bars

Preparation Time: 15 minutes **Chilling Time:** 2 hours **Difficulty:** Easy **Servings:** 12 bars

Ingredients:

- 1 cup almonds
- 1 cup pitted dates
- 1/4 cup unsweetened cocoa powder
- Optional toppings: shredded coconut, chopped almonds
- 2 tablespoons almond butter
- 2 tablespoons honey or maple syrup
- 1 teaspoon vanilla extract
- Pinch of salt

Instructions:

1. Place the almonds in a food processor and pulse until they are finely chopped.
2. Add the pitted dates, cocoa powder, almond butter, honey or maple syrup, vanilla extract, and salt to the food processor. Process until the mixture forms a sticky dough.
3. Line an 8x8-inch baking dish with parchment paper or lightly grease it with cooking spray.
4. Transfer the almond date mixture into the prepared baking dish. Use a spatula or your hands to press the mixture firmly and evenly into the dish.
5. If desired, sprinkle shredded coconut or chopped almonds on top of the mixture and press them gently to adhere.
6. Place the dish in the refrigerator and chill for at least 2 hours to firm up.
7. Once chilled, remove the mixture from the dish and cut it into 12 bars.
8. Individually wrap the bars in plastic wrap or store them in an airtight container in the refrigerator for up to 2 weeks.

Nutritional Information (per bar):

Calories: 145

Fat: 7.2g

Saturated Fat: 0.6g

Trans Fat: 0g

Cholesterol: 0mg

Sodium: 1mg

Carbohydrates: 19.9g

Fiber: 3.6g

Sugar: 15.7g

Protein: 3.3g

Vitamin D: 0mcg

Calcium: 41mg

Iron: 1mg

Potassium: 232mg

savory muffins with peas and ham

Preparation Time: 15 minutes **Cooking Time:** 20 minutes **Difficulty:** Easy **Servings:** 12 muffins

Ingredients:

- 2 cups all-purpose flour
- 2 teaspoons baking powder
- 1/2 teaspoon baking soda
- 1/2 teaspoon salt
- 1/4 teaspoon black pepper
- 1/2 cup cooked peas (fresh or frozen)
- 1/2 cup diced cooked ham
- 1/4 cup grated cheddar cheese
- 2 green onions, finely chopped
- 1/4 cup chopped fresh parsley
- 1 cup buttermilk
- 1/4 cup vegetable oil
- 2 large eggs

Instructions:

1. Preheat the oven to 375°F (190°C). Grease or line a 12-cup muffin tin with paper liners.
2. In a large bowl, whisk together the flour, baking powder, baking soda, salt, and black pepper.
3. Add the cooked peas, diced ham, grated cheddar cheese, green onions, and chopped parsley to the dry ingredients. Stir to combine.
4. In a separate bowl, whisk together the buttermilk, vegetable oil, and eggs.
5. Pour the wet ingredients into the dry ingredients. Stir until just combined. Be careful not to overmix; the batter should be slightly lumpy.
6. Divide the batter evenly among the prepared muffin cups, filling each about three-quarters full.
7. Bake for 18-20 minutes, or until a toothpick inserted into the center of a muffin comes out clean.

8. Remove the muffins from the oven and let them cool in the tin for a few minutes. Then transfer them to a wire rack to cool completely.

Nutritional Information (per muffin)

Calories: 171
Fat: 7.1g
Saturated Fat: 2g
Trans Fat: 0g
Cholesterol: 32mg

Sodium: 402mg
Carbohydrates: 20.9g
Fiber: 1g
Sugar: 1.7g
Protein: 6.7g

Savory herb pancakes

Preparation Time: 10 minutes **Cooking Time:** 15 minutes **Difficulty:** Easy **Servings:** 4 pancakes

Ingredients:

- 1 cup all-purpose flour
- 1 teaspoon baking powder
- 1/2 teaspoon salt
- 1/4 teaspoon black pepper
- 1 tablespoon chopped fresh herbs (such as parsley, chives, or basil)
- 1/2 cup milk
- 1/4 cup plain Greek yogurt
- 1 large egg
- 2 tablespoons melted butter or olive oil
- Additional butter or oil for cooking

Instructions:

1. In a large bowl, whisk together the flour, baking powder, salt, black pepper, and chopped fresh herbs.
2. In a separate bowl, whisk together the milk, Greek yogurt, egg, and melted butter or olive oil.
3. Pour the wet ingredients into the dry ingredients. Stir until just combined. The batter should be slightly lumpy.
4. Heat a non-stick skillet or griddle over medium heat. Add a small amount of butter or oil to the skillet and spread it evenly.
5. Spoon about 1/4 cup of the batter onto the skillet for each pancake. Use the back of the spoon to spread the batter into a round shape.
6. Cook the pancakes for 2-3 minutes, or until bubbles form on the surface. Flip the pancakes and cook for an additional 1-2 minutes, or until golden brown and cooked through.
7. Transfer the cooked pancakes to a plate and cover with a clean kitchen towel to keep them warm.
8. Repeat steps 5-7 with the remaining batter, adding more butter or oil to the skillet as needed.

Nutritional Information (per pancake):

Calories: 192
Fat: 9g
Saturated Fat: 5g
Trans Fat: 0g
Cholesterol: 67mg
Sodium: 437mg
Carbohydrates: 21g
Fiber: 1g
Sugar: 1g
Protein: 7g

Salted Caramel Cheesecake

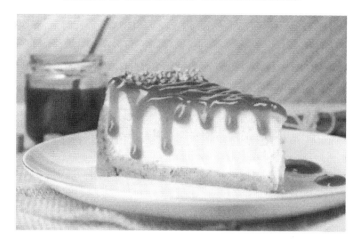

Preparation Time:

30 minutes **Chilling Time:** 4 hours or overnight **Baking Time:** 1 hour **Difficulty:** Intermediate **Servings:** 12-16 slices

Ingredients:

For the Crust:

- 2 cups graham cracker crumbs
- 1/4 cup granulated sugar
- 1/2 cup unsalted butter, melted

For the Cheesecake Filling:

- 24 oz (680g) cream cheese, softened
- 1 cup granulated sugar
- 3 large eggs

- 1 tsp vanilla extract

For the Salted Caramel Sauce:

- 1 cup granulated sugar
- 6 tbsp unsalted butter, room temperature
- 1/2 cup heavy cream
- 1 tsp sea salt (adjust to taste)

For the Topping:

- Whipped cream (optional)
- Additional salted caramel sauce (optional)

Instructions:

1. Preheat your oven to 325°F (160°C). Grease the bottom of a 9-inch (23cm) springform pan and line it with parchment paper.
2. In a mixing bowl, combine the graham cracker crumbs, granulated sugar, and melted butter for the crust. Stir until the mixture resembles wet sand.
3. Press the crust mixture firmly into the bottom of the prepared springform pan, forming an even layer. Set aside.
4. In a large mixing bowl, beat the softened cream cheese and granulated sugar until smooth and creamy. Add the eggs one at a time, beating well after each addition. Stir in the vanilla extract.
5. Pour the cheesecake filling over the prepared crust in the springform pan. Smooth the top with a spatula.
6. Place the springform pan on a baking sheet and bake in the preheated oven for about 1 hour, or until the edges are set and the center is slightly jiggly.
7. Remove the cheesecake from the oven and let it cool in the pan for 10 minutes. Then, run a knife around the edges to loosen it from the pan. Allow it to cool completely on a wire rack.
8. While the cheesecake is cooling, prepare the salted caramel sauce. In a saucepan, heat the granulated sugar over medium heat, stirring constantly until it melts and turns amber in color.
9. Add the butter to the caramelized sugar, stirring until melted and well combined. Remove the saucepan from heat and carefully pour in the heavy cream, stirring constantly.
10. Return the saucepan to low heat and cook for another 2 minutes, stirring continuously, until the caramel sauce thickens slightly. Stir in the sea salt, adjusting the amount to your desired level of saltiness.
11. Pour the salted caramel sauce over the cooled cheesecake, spreading it evenly with a spatula. Reserve some sauce for drizzling on top.
12. Place the cheesecake in the refrigerator and let it chill for at least 4 hours or overnight to set.
13. Before serving, remove the sides of the springform pan. If desired, pipe some whipped cream around the edges and drizzle with additional salted caramel sauce.

Nutritional values:

Calories: 531
Fat: 35g
Saturated Fat: 20g
Trans Fat: 1g
Cholesterol: 143mg

Sodium: 481mg
Carbohydrates: 49g
Fiber: 0g
Sugar: 41g
Protein: 7g

Savoury Basil Biscuits

Preparation Time:

15 minutes **Cooking Time:** 15 minutes **Difficulty:** Easy **Servings:** 12 biscuits

Ingredients:

- 2 cups whole wheat flour
- 1 tablespoon baking powder
- 1/2 teaspoon salt
- 1/4 teaspoon black pepper
- 1/4 cup chopped fresh basil
- 1/4 cup grated Parmesan cheese
- 1/4 cup unsalted butter, cold and cut into small pieces
- 3/4 cup skim milk

Instructions:

1. Preheat your oven to 425°F (220°C). Line a baking sheet with parchment paper or lightly grease it with cooking spray.
2. In a large bowl, whisk together the whole wheat flour, baking powder, salt, black pepper, chopped fresh basil, and grated Parmesan cheese.
3. Add the cold butter pieces to the flour mixture. Use a pastry cutter or your fingers to cut the butter into the flour until the mixture resembles coarse crumbs.
4. Gradually pour in the skim milk and stir until the dough comes together. Be careful not to overmix.
5. Transfer the dough onto a lightly floured surface and gently knead it a few times to bring it together.
6. Roll out the dough to a 1/2-inch thickness. Use a round biscuit cutter or a glass to cut out biscuits from the dough. Place the biscuits onto the prepared baking sheet.
7. Bake the biscuits in the preheated oven for 12-15 minutes, or until they are golden brown and cooked through.
8. Remove the biscuits from the oven and transfer them to a wire rack to cool slightly before serving.

Nutritional Information (per biscuit):

Calories: 128
Fat: 4g
Saturated Fat: 2g
Trans Fat: 0g
Cholesterol: 9mg

Sodium: 272mg
Carbohydrates: 19g
Fiber: 3g
Sugar: 1g
Protein: 5g

Stuffed Mushrooms

Preparation Time: 15 minutes **Cooking Time**: 20-25 minutes **Difficulty**: Easy **Servings**: 4

Ingredients:

- 16 large button mushrooms, stems removed
- 1/2 cup cooked quinoa
- 1/4 cup chopped walnuts
- 1/4 cup chopped sun-dried tomatoes
- 1/4 cup chopped fresh parsley
- 1/4 cup chopped fresh basil
- 2 cloves garlic, minced
- 2 tbsp olive oil
- Salt and pepper to taste

Instructions:

1. Preheat the oven to 375°F (190°C).
2. Clean the mushrooms and remove their stems. Set the mushroom caps aside.
3. In a mixing bowl, combine the quinoa, walnuts, sun-dried tomatoes, parsley, basil, garlic, olive oil, salt, and pepper. Mix well.
4. Stuff each mushroom cap with the quinoa mixture.
5. Place the stuffed mushrooms on a baking sheet and bake for 20-25 minutes, until the mushrooms are tender and the filling is golden brown.
6. Serve hot.

Nutritional Information (per serving):

Calories: 129
Total Fat: 10g
Saturated Fat: 1g
Cholesterol: 0mg
Sodium: 16mg

Total Carbohydrates: 9g
Dietary Fiber: 2g
Sugars: 2g
Protein: 4g

Zucchini Quiche

Preparation Time: 15 minutes **Cooking Time:** 40 minutes **Difficulty:** Intermediate **Servings:** 6

Ingredients:

- 1 pre-made pie crust
- 2 medium zucchinis, thinly sliced
- 1 small onion, diced
- 1 clove garlic, minced
- 1 tablespoon olive oil
- 4 large eggs
- 1 cup milk (any type, such as whole, skim, or plant-based)
- 1 cup shredded cheese (such as cheddar, mozzarella, or Swiss)
- Salt and pepper to taste
- Fresh herbs for garnish (optional)

Instructions:

1. Preheat your oven to 375°F (190°C). Place the pre-made pie crust into a 9-inch (23cm) pie dish and set it aside.
2. In a large skillet, heat the olive oil over medium heat. Add the diced onion and minced garlic, and sauté until the onion becomes translucent and fragrant, about 2-3 minutes.
3. Add the thinly sliced zucchini to the skillet and continue to cook for another 3-4 minutes, until the zucchini becomes tender. Remove from heat and set aside.
4. In a mixing bowl, whisk together the eggs, milk, salt, and pepper until well combined.
5. Spread the cooked zucchini mixture evenly over the pre-made pie crust in the pie dish. Sprinkle the shredded cheese over the zucchini.
6. Pour the egg mixture over the zucchini and cheese, ensuring it fills the pie crust evenly.
7. Place the quiche in the preheated oven and bake for 35-40 minutes, or until the center is set and the top is golden brown.
8. Once baked, remove the quiche from the oven and let it cool for a few minutes. Slice into wedges and serve warm.

Nutritional Information (per serving):

Calories: 297
Total Fat: 19g
Saturated Fat: 7g
Cholesterol: 132mg
Sodium: 359mg

Total Carbohydrates: 18g
Dietary Fiber: 1g
Sugars: 4g
Protein: 13g

Eggplant Savory Pie

Preparation Time: 30 minutes **Cooking Time**: 45 minutes **Difficulty**: Intermediate **Servings**: 6

Ingredients:

- 1 pre-made pie crust
- 2 medium aubergines (eggplants), thinly sliced
- 1 medium onion, diced
- 2 cloves garlic, minced
- 2 tablespoons olive oil
- 1 cup diced tomatoes (fresh or canned)
- 1 tablespoon tomato paste
- 1 teaspoon dried oregano
- 1/2 teaspoon dried basil
- 1/2 teaspoon dried thyme
- Salt and pepper to taste
- 1 cup shredded cheese (such as mozzarella or feta)
- Fresh basil leaves for garnish (optional)

Instructions:

1. Preheat your oven to 375°F (190°C). Place the pre-made pie crust into a 9-inch (23cm) pie dish and set it aside.
2. Heat the olive oil in a large skillet over medium heat. Add the diced onion and minced garlic, and sauté until the onion becomes translucent and fragrant, about 2-3 minutes.
3. Add the sliced aubergines to the skillet and cook until they become tender, about 8-10 minutes. Stir occasionally to prevent sticking.
4. Add the diced tomatoes, tomato paste, dried oregano, dried basil, dried thyme, salt, and pepper to the skillet. Stir well to combine all the ingredients. Cook for an additional 2-3 minutes to allow the flavors to meld.
5. Remove the skillet from heat and let the mixture cool slightly.
6. Spread the aubergine mixture evenly over the pre-made pie crust in the pie dish.
7. Sprinkle the shredded cheese over the top of the aubergine mixture.
8. Place the pie dish in the preheated oven and bake for 35-45 minutes, or until the crust is golden brown and the cheese has melted.
9. Once baked, remove the pie from the oven and let it cool for a few minutes. Garnish with fresh basil leaves, if desired.
10. Slice into wedges and serve warm.

Nutritional Information (per serving):

Calories: 285
Total Fat: 15g
Saturated Fat: 5g
Cholesterol: 19mg
Sodium: 385mg

Total Carbohydrates: 29g
Dietary Fiber: 5g
Sugars: 7g
Protein: 9g

Green Detox Smoothie

Preparation time: 5 minutes **Serving size**: 1

Ingredients:

- 1 cup spinach
- 1/2 cucumber, peeled and chopped
- 1/2 lemon, juiced
- 1 cup coconut water
- 1/2 green apple, cored and chopped
- 1/2 ripe avocado
- Ice cubes (optional)

Nutritional values (per serving):

Calories: 150
Carbohydrates: 20g
Fat: 7g

Protein: 4g
Fiber: 7g
Sugar: 9g

Berry Protein Smoothie

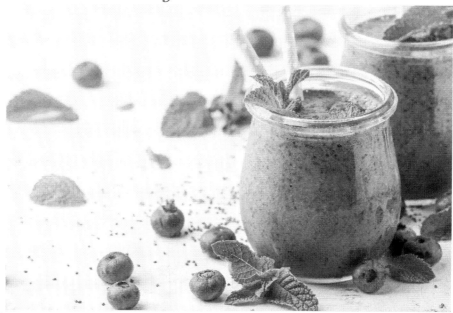

Preparation time: 5 minutes **Serving size:** 1

Ingredients:

- 1 cup mixed berries (strawberries, blueberries, raspberries)
- 1/2 ripe banana
- 1 scoop plant-based protein powder
- 1 cup almond milk
- 1 tablespoon chia seeds (optional)
- Ice cubes

Nutritional values (per serving):

Calories: 240

Carbohydrates: 35g

Fat: 6g

Protein: 18g

Fiber: 10g

Sugar: 15g

Tropical Mango Smoothie

Preparation time: 5 minutes **Serving size:** 1

Ingredients:

- 1 ripe mango, peeled and chopped
- 1/2 cup pineapple chunks
- 1/2 cup coconut milk
- 1/2 cup Greek yogurt
- 1 tablespoon honey (optional)
- Ice cubes

Nutritional values (per serving):

Calories: 270

Carbohydrates: 49g

Fat: 5g

Protein: 11g

Fiber: 5g

Sugar: 41g

Purple Sweet Potato Smoothie

Preparation time: 10 minutes **Serving size:** 1

Ingredients:

- 1 small purple sweet potato, cooked and peeled
- 1/2 cup frozen blueberries
- 1/2 ripe banana
- 1 cup almond milk
- 1 tablespoon honey or maple syrup (optional)
- 1/2 teaspoon vanilla extract
- Ice cubes

Instructions:

1. Cook the purple sweet potato by boiling or roasting it until tender. Let it cool, then peel the skin off.
2. In a blender, combine the cooked sweet potato, frozen blueberries, ripe banana, almond milk, honey or maple syrup (if using), and vanilla extract.
3. Blend until smooth and creamy.
4. If the smoothie is too thick, add more almond milk or water to reach your desired consistency.
5. Add a few ice cubes and blend again until well incorporated.
6. Pour the smoothie into a glass and enjoy the unique flavors and vibrant purple color!

Nutritional values (per serving):

Calories: 250

Carbohydrates: 54g

Fat: 3g

Protein: 4g

Fiber: 8g

Sugar: 23g

Apple, Pear, and Cinnamon Smoothie

Preparation time: 5 minutes Serving size: 1

Ingredients:

- 1 medium apple, cored and chopped
- 1 medium pear, cored and chopped
- 1/2 cup unsweetened applesauce
- 1 cup almond milk (or any milk of your choice)
- 1 tablespoon honey or maple syrup (optional)
- 1/2 teaspoon ground cinnamon
- Ice cubes

Instructions:

1. In a blender, combine the chopped apple, chopped pear, unsweetened applesauce, almond milk, honey or maple syrup (if using), and ground cinnamon.
2. Blend until smooth and creamy.
3. If the smoothie is too thick, add more almond milk or water to reach your desired consistency.
4. Add a few ice cubes and blend again until well incorporated.
5. Taste and adjust the sweetness or cinnamon level if desired.
6. Pour the smoothie into a glass and sprinkle some extra ground cinnamon on top for garnish.
7. Enjoy the comforting flavors of apple, pear, and cinnamon in this delicious smoothie!

Nutritional values (per serving):

- Calories: 190
- Carbohydrates: 46g
- Fat: 2g
- Protein: 2g
- Fiber: 8g
- Sugar: 32g

Cappuccino Smoothie

Preparation time: 5 minutes Serving size: 1
Ingredients:

- 1 cup brewed coffee, chilled
- 1 ripe banana
- 1/2 cup unsweetened almond milk (or any milk of your choice)
- 1 tablespoon almond butter or peanut butter
- 1 tablespoon cocoa powder
- 1 tablespoon honey or maple syrup (optional)
- 1/2 teaspoon vanilla extract
- Ice cubes

Instructions:

1. In a blender, combine the chilled brewed coffee, ripe banana, almond milk, almond butter or peanut butter, cocoa powder, honey or maple syrup (if using), and vanilla extract.
2. Blend until smooth and creamy.
3. If the smoothie is too thick, add more almond milk or water to reach your desired consistency.
4. Add a few ice cubes and blend again until well incorporated.
5. Taste and adjust the sweetness or coffee intensity if desired.
6. Pour the smoothie into a glass and sprinkle some cocoa powder on top for garnish.
7. Enjoy the rich and indulgent flavors of a cappuccino in this delightful smoothie!

Nutritional values (per serving):

Calories: 220
Carbohydrates: 38g
Fat: 7g
Protein: 5g
Fiber: 6g
Sugar: 20g

Energy Balls

Preparation time: 15 minutes Serving size: 10-12 balls
Ingredients:

- 1 cup rolled oats
- 1/2 cup nut butter (e.g., almond butter, peanut butter)
- 1/4 cup honey or maple syrup
- 1/4 cup ground flaxseed
- 1/4 cup mini chocolate chips
- 1/4 cup dried fruits (e.g., cranberries, raisins)
- 1 teaspoon vanilla extract

Instructions:

1. In a mixing bowl, combine all the ingredients.
2. Mix well until all the ingredients are evenly distributed.
3. Roll the mixture into small balls using your hands.
4. Place the balls on a baking sheet and refrigerate for at least 1 hour to firm up.
5. Once firm, store the energy balls in an airtight container in the refrigerator.

Nutritional values (per serving, based on 12 balls):

Calories: 160
Carbohydrates: 19g
Fat: 8g
Protein: 4g
Fiber: 3g
Sugar: 9g

Veggie Sticks with Hummus

Preparation time: 10 minutes Serving size: 2-4

Ingredients:

- Assorted vegetables (carrot sticks, celery sticks, bell pepper strips, cucumber slices, etc.)
- Hummus for dipping

Instructions:

1. Wash and cut the vegetables into sticks or slices.
2. Arrange the veggie sticks on a platter.
3. Serve with a bowl of hummus for dipping.
4. Enjoy this refreshing and nutritious snack packed with vitamins and fiber!

Nutritional values (per serving, based on 2-4 servings):

Calories: 70-140

Carbohydrates: 10-20g

Fat: 3-7g

Protein: 3-6g

Fiber: 3-5g

Sugar: 3-5g

Baked Kale Chips

Preparation time: 15 minutes Cooking time: 15 minutes Serving size: 2-4

Ingredients:

- 1 bunch of kale, washed and dried
- 1 tablespoon olive oil
- Salt, to taste
- Optional seasonings: garlic powder, paprika, chili flakes, etc.

Instructions:

1. Preheat your oven to 350°F (175°C).
2. Remove the tough stems from the kale leaves and tear them into bite-sized pieces.
3. In a large bowl, drizzle the kale with olive oil and sprinkle with salt and any desired seasonings.
4. Massage the oil and seasonings into the kale leaves until well coated.
5. Arrange the kale pieces in a single layer on a baking sheet lined with parchment paper.
6. Bake for 10-15 minutes, or until the kale chips are crispy and slightly browned.

Nutritional values (per serving, based on 2-4 servings):

Calories: 50-100

Carbohydrates: 7-15g

Fat: 2-4g

Protein: 3-5g

Fiber: 2-4g

Sugar: 1-2g

DESSERT RECIPES
Sweet Beetroot Cake

Preparation time: 20 minutes Cooking time: 45 minutes Difficulty: Intermediate Servings: 8-10

Ingredients:

- 2 cups grated beetroot
- 1 ½ cups whole wheat flour
- ½ cup almond flour
- ½ cup unsweetened applesauce
- ½ cup maple syrup or honey
- ¼ cup olive oil
- 3 large eggs
- 1 teaspoon vanilla extract
- 1 teaspoon baking powder
- 1 teaspoon ground cinnamon
- ½ teaspoon ground nutmeg
- ¼ teaspoon salt
- Optional toppings: powdered sugar, fresh berries

Instructions:

1. Preheat the oven to 350°F (175°C). Grease and flour a round cake pan.
2. In a large mixing bowl, combine the grated beetroot, whole wheat flour, almond flour, baking powder, ground cinnamon, ground nutmeg, and salt. Mix well.
3. In a separate bowl, whisk together the applesauce, maple syrup or honey, olive oil, eggs, and vanilla extract until well combined.
4. Gradually add the wet ingredients to the dry ingredients, stirring until just combined. Do not overmix.
5. Pour the batter into the prepared cake pan and smooth the top with a spatula.
6. Bake for 40-45 minutes, or until a toothpick inserted into the center comes out clean.
7. Remove the cake from the oven and let it cool in the pan for 10 minutes. Then transfer it to a wire rack to cool completely.
8. Once cooled, you can sprinkle powdered sugar on top and decorate with fresh berries if desired.

Nutritional values (per serving):

Calories: 220

Carbohydrates: 30g

Fat: 9g

Protein: 5g

Fiber: 4g

Sugar: 15g

Lemon Blueberry Cake

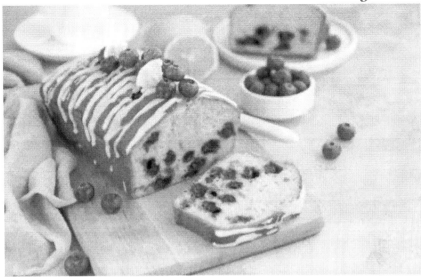

Preparation time: 20 minutes Cooking time: 40 minutes Difficulty: Intermediate Servings: 8-10

Ingredients: For the cake:

- 1 ½ cups whole wheat flour
- ½ cup almond flour
- 1 teaspoon baking powder
- ½ teaspoon baking soda
- ¼ teaspoon salt
- ½ cup unsweetened applesauce
- ½ cup maple syrup or honey
- ¼ cup olive oil
- ¼ cup fresh lemon juice
- 2 tablespoons lemon zest
- 2 large eggs
- 1 teaspoon vanilla extract
- 1 cup fresh or frozen blueberries

For the lemon glaze:

- ½ cup powdered sugar
- 2 tablespoons fresh lemon juice
- 1 tablespoon lemon zest

Instructions:

1. Preheat the oven to 350°F (175°C). Grease and flour a round cake pan.
2. In a mixing bowl, whisk together the whole wheat flour, almond flour, baking powder, baking soda, and salt.
3. In a separate bowl, combine the applesauce, maple syrup or honey, olive oil, lemon juice, lemon zest, eggs, and vanilla extract. Mix well.
4. Gradually add the wet ingredients to the dry ingredients, stirring until just combined. Avoid overmixing.
5. Gently fold in the blueberries.
6. Pour the batter into the prepared cake pan and smooth the top with a spatula.
7. Bake for 35-40 minutes, or until a toothpick inserted into the center comes out clean.
8. While the cake is baking, prepare the lemon glaze by whisking together the powdered sugar, lemon juice, and lemon zest until smooth.
9. Once the cake is done, remove it from the oven and let it cool in the pan for 10 minutes. Then transfer it to a wire rack.
10. Drizzle the lemon glaze over the cooled cake, allowing it to drizzle down the sides.
11. Slice and serve this tangy and refreshing Lemon Blueberry Cake, perfect for any special occasion or as a delightful treat!

Nutritional values (per serving):

Calories: 240

Carbohydrates: 35g

Fat: 9g

Protein: 4g

Fiber: 3g

Sugar: 18g

Pumpkin Fritters

Preparation time: 15 minutes Cooking time: 15 minutes Difficulty: Easy Servings: 4
Ingredients:

- 1 cup pumpkin puree
- 1/2 cup whole wheat flour
- 1/4 cup almond flour
- 1 teaspoon baking powder
- 1/2 teaspoon ground cinnamon
- 1/4 teaspoon ground nutmeg
- 1/4 teaspoon salt
- 1 tablespoon maple syrup or honey
- 1/2 teaspoon vanilla extract
- 1 tablespoon unsweetened almond milk (or any non-dairy milk)
- Cooking oil for frying
- Optional toppings: powdered sugar, cinnamon, or maple syrup

Instructions:

1. In a large mixing bowl, combine the pumpkin puree, whole wheat flour, almond flour, baking powder, cinnamon, nutmeg, salt, maple syrup or honey, vanilla extract, and almond milk. Stir well until a thick batter forms.
2. Heat a skillet or frying pan over medium heat and add enough cooking oil to cover the bottom.
3. Drop spoonfuls of the pumpkin batter onto the hot skillet, using approximately 2 tablespoons of batter for each fritter.
4. Cook the fritters for 3-4 minutes on each side, or until they turn golden brown. Flip them carefully using a spatula.
5. Once cooked, transfer the fritters to a plate lined with paper towels to absorb any excess oil.
6. Repeat the process with the remaining batter, adding more oil to the pan as needed.
7. Serve the Pumpkin Fritters warm. You can dust them with powdered sugar and sprinkle with cinnamon or drizzle with maple syrup for extra flavor.

Nutritional values (per serving, without toppings):

Calories: 140
Carbohydrates: 25g
Fat: 3g

Protein: 4g
Fiber: 4g
Sugar: 7g

Coconut Milk Rolls

Preparation time: 2 hours 30 minutes (including rising time) Cooking time: 20 minutes Difficulty: Intermediate Servings: 12 rolls
Ingredients: For the rolls:

- 2 3/4 cups all-purpose flour
- 2 tablespoons granulated sugar
- 1 teaspoon salt
- 2 1/4 teaspoons instant yeast
- 1/2 cup coconut milk
- 1/4 cup water
- 2 tablespoons coconut oil, melted
- 1 teaspoon vanilla extract

For the coconut filling:

- 1/2 cup shredded coconut
- 1/4 cup granulated sugar
- 2 tablespoons coconut oil, melted

For the glaze:

- 1/2 cup powdered sugar
- 1-2 tablespoons coconut milk

Instructions:

1. In a large mixing bowl, combine the all-purpose flour, sugar, salt, and instant yeast.
2. In a separate microwave-safe bowl, heat the coconut milk and water together until warm (about 110°F or 43°C).
3. Pour the warm coconut milk mixture, melted coconut oil, and vanilla extract into the dry ingredients. Stir until a dough forms.
4. Transfer the dough onto a floured surface and knead for about 5 minutes until smooth and elastic.
5. Place the dough in a greased bowl, cover with a clean kitchen towel, and let it rise in a warm place for about 1 hour, or until doubled in size.
6. In the meantime, prepare the coconut filling. In a small bowl, mix together the shredded coconut, granulated sugar, and melted coconut oil. Set aside.

7. Once the dough has doubled in size, punch it down and turn it out onto a floured surface. Roll it out into a rectangle, about 1/4 inch thick.
8. Spread the coconut filling evenly over the dough, leaving a small border around the edges.
9. Starting from one long side, tightly roll up the dough into a log. Pinch the seam to seal.
10. Cut the log into 12 equal-sized rolls using a sharp knife or dental floss.
11. Place the rolls in a greased baking dish, cover with a kitchen towel, and let them rise for another 1 hour, or until puffed and doubled in size.
12. Preheat the oven to 375°F (190°C).
13. Bake the rolls for 18-20 minutes, or until golden brown and cooked through.
14. While the rolls are baking, prepare the glaze by whisking together the powdered sugar and coconut milk until smooth.
15. Once the rolls are out of the oven, drizzle them with the glaze.
16. Allow the Coconut Milk Rolls to cool slightly before serving.

Nutritional values (per serving):

Calories: 225

Carbohydrates: 35g

Fat: 8g

Protein: 4g

Fiber: 2g

Sugar: 9g

Tiramisu

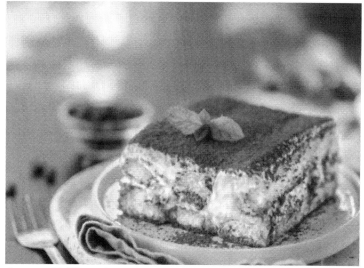

Preparation time: 30 minutes Chilling time: 4 hours or overnight Difficulty: Intermediate Servings: 8

Ingredients:

- 24 ladyfinger cookies
- 1 1/2 cups strong brewed coffee, cooled
- 1/4 cup rum (optional)
- 8 ounces mascarpone cheese
- 1/2 cup powdered sugar

- 1 teaspoon vanilla extract
- 1 cup heavy cream
- 2 tablespoons unsweetened cocoa powder, for dusting

Instructions:

1. In a shallow dish, combine the cooled brewed coffee and rum (if using).
2. In a mixing bowl, beat the mascarpone cheese, powdered sugar, and vanilla extract until smooth.
3. In a separate bowl, whip the heavy cream until soft peaks form.
4. Gently fold the whipped cream into the mascarpone mixture until well combined.
5. Dip each ladyfinger cookie into the coffee mixture for a few seconds, making sure not to oversoak them.
6. Arrange a layer of soaked ladyfingers in the bottom of an 8x8-inch dish or individual serving glasses.
7. Spread half of the mascarpone mixture over the ladyfingers.
8. Repeat with another layer of soaked ladyfingers and the remaining mascarpone mixture.
9. Sift cocoa powder over the top to evenly dust the surface.
10. Cover the dish with plastic wrap and refrigerate for at least 4 hours or overnight to allow the flavors to meld and the dessert to set.
11. Prior to serving, you can dust an additional layer of cocoa powder on top for presentation if desired.
12. Serve chilled.

Nutritional values (per serving):

Calories: 350
Carbohydrates: 28g
Fat: 24g

Protein: 5g
Fiber: 1g
Sugar: 11g

Pistachio Biscuits

Preparation time: 20 minutes Cooking time: 12-15 minutes Difficulty: Easy Servings: 20 biscuits

Ingredients:

- 1 cup shelled pistachios
- 1 1/4 cups all-purpose flour
- 1/2 cup unsalted butter, softened
- 1/2 cup granulated sugar
- 1/2 teaspoon vanilla extract
- 1/4 teaspoon almond extract (optional)
- 1/4 teaspoon salt
- 1 egg yolk
- Extra pistachios for decoration (optional)

Instructions:

1. Preheat the oven to 350°F (175°C). Line a baking sheet with parchment paper.
2. In a food processor, pulse the shelled pistachios until finely ground. Set aside.
3. In a mixing bowl, cream together the softened butter and granulated sugar until light and fluffy.
4. Add the vanilla extract, almond extract (if using), and salt to the butter-sugar mixture. Mix well.
5. Gradually add the ground pistachios and flour to the mixture. Mix until the dough comes together.
6. Roll the dough into small balls, about 1 inch in diameter. Place them on the prepared baking sheet, leaving some space between each biscuit.
7. Flatten each ball slightly with the back of a fork, creating a crisscross pattern on top.
8. Optional: Press a pistachio into the center of each biscuit for decoration.
9. In a small bowl, lightly beat the egg yolk. Brush the top of each biscuit with the beaten egg yolk.
10. Bake the biscuits in the preheated oven for 12-15 minutes, or until the edges turn golden brown.
11. Remove from the oven and let the biscuits cool on the baking sheet for a few minutes before transferring them to a wire rack to cool completely.

Nutritional values (per biscuit):

Calories: 100

Carbohydrates: 8g

Fat: 7g

Protein: 2g

Fiber: 1g

Sugar: 4g

Almond Biscuits with Chocolate Drizzle

Preparation time: 20 minutes Cooking time: 12-15 minutes Difficulty: Easy Servings: 24 biscuits

Ingredients:

- 1 1/2 cups almond flour
- 1/2 cup granulated sugar
- 1/4 cup unsalted butter, softened
- 1/2 teaspoon almond extract
- 1/4 teaspoon salt
- 1 egg
- 1/4 cup sliced almonds
- 2 ounces dark chocolate, melted

Instructions:

1. Preheat the oven to 350°F (175°C). Line a baking sheet with parchment paper.
2. In a mixing bowl, combine the almond flour, granulated sugar, softened butter, almond extract, and salt. Mix well until the ingredients are evenly incorporated.
3. Add the egg to the mixture and continue mixing until a dough forms.
4. Roll the dough into small balls, about 1 inch in diameter. Place them on the prepared baking sheet, leaving some space between each biscuit.
5. Flatten each ball slightly with the palm of your hand and press a few sliced almonds onto the top of each biscuit.
6. Bake the biscuits in the preheated oven for 12-15 minutes, or until the edges turn golden brown.
7. Remove from the oven and let the biscuits cool on the baking sheet for a few minutes before transferring them to a wire rack to cool completely.
8. Once the biscuits are cooled, drizzle the melted dark chocolate over the top of each biscuit.
9. Allow the chocolate to set before serving or storing the biscuits.

Nutritional values (per biscuit):

Calories: 90

Carbohydrates: 6g

Fat: 7g

Protein: 2g

Fiber: 1g

Sugar: 4g

Chocolate Cake with a Dark Heart

Preparation time: 20 minutes Cooking time: 30-35 minutes Difficulty: Intermediate Servings: 10-12

Ingredients: For the cake:

- 1 3/4 cups all-purpose flour
- 1 1/2 cups granulated sugar
- 3/4 cup unsweetened cocoa powder
- 1 1/2 teaspoons baking powder
- 1 1/2 teaspoons baking soda
- 1 teaspoon salt
- 2 large eggs
- 1 cup milk
- 1/2 cup vegetable oil

- 2 teaspoons vanilla extract
- 1 cup boiling water

For the dark heart filling:

- 4 ounces dark chocolate, chopped
- 1/2 cup heavy cream

For the frosting:

- 1 1/2 cups heavy cream
- 1/4 cup powdered sugar
- 1 teaspoon vanilla extract

Instructions:

1. Preheat the oven to 350°F (175°C). Grease and flour two 9-inch round cake pans.
2. In a large mixing bowl, whisk together the flour, sugar, cocoa powder, baking powder, baking soda, and salt.
3. Add the eggs, milk, vegetable oil, and vanilla extract to the dry ingredients. Mix until well combined.
4. Gradually pour in the boiling water while stirring continuously. The batter will be thin, but that's normal.
5. Divide the batter evenly between the prepared cake pans.
6. In a small saucepan, heat the heavy cream for the dark heart filling until it just begins to simmer. Remove from heat and pour over the chopped dark chocolate. Let it sit for a minute, then stir until smooth and well combined.
7. Spoon the dark chocolate filling onto the center of one cake batter in a heart shape.
8. Carefully place the second cake batter over the filling, making sure to cover the heart completely.
9. Bake in the preheated oven for 30-35 minutes, or until a toothpick inserted into the center comes out clean.
10. Remove from the oven and let the cakes cool in the pans for 10 minutes before transferring them to a wire rack to cool completely.
11. In a mixing bowl, whip the heavy cream for the frosting until soft peaks form. Add the powdered sugar and vanilla extract, and continue whipping until stiff peaks form.
12. Place one cake layer on a serving plate and spread a generous amount of whipped cream frosting on top. Place the second cake layer on top and frost the entire cake with the remaining whipped cream.
13. Optional: Decorate the cake with chocolate shavings, sprinkles, or fresh berries.

Nutritional values (per serving):

Calories: 400

Carbohydrates: 47g

Fat: 24g

Protein: 5g

Fiber: 3g

Sugar: 32g

Apple and Vanilla Cake

Preparation time: 20 minutes Cooking time: 45-50 minutes Difficulty: Easy Servings: 10-12

Ingredients:

- 2 cups all-purpose flour
- 1 1/2 teaspoons baking powder
- 1/2 teaspoon baking soda
- 1/2 teaspoon salt
- 1 teaspoon ground cinnamon
- 1/2 cup unsalted butter, softened
- 1 cup granulated sugar
- 2 large eggs
- 1 teaspoon vanilla extract
- 1/2 cup milk
- 2 cups peeled, cored, and diced apples (about 2 medium-sized apples)
- Powdered sugar for dusting (optional)

Instructions:

1. Preheat the oven to 350°F (175°C). Grease and flour a 9-inch round cake pan.
2. In a mixing bowl, whisk together the flour, baking powder, baking soda, salt, and ground cinnamon. Set aside.
3. In a separate large mixing bowl, cream together the softened butter and granulated sugar until light and fluffy.
4. Add the eggs, one at a time, beating well after each addition. Stir in the vanilla extract.
5. Gradually add the dry ingredients to the butter mixture, alternating with the milk. Begin and end with the dry ingredients, mixing just until combined.
6. Gently fold in the diced apples until evenly distributed throughout the batter.
7. Pour the batter into the prepared cake pan and smooth the top with a spatula.
8. Bake in the preheated oven for 45-50 minutes, or until a toothpick inserted into the center comes out clean.
9. Remove from the oven and let the cake cool in the pan for 10 minutes. Then transfer it to a wire rack to cool completely.
10. Optional: Dust the top of the cooled cake with powdered sugar for a decorative touch.

Nutritional values (per serving):

Calories: 250
Carbohydrates: 36g
Fat: 10g

Protein: 3g
Fiber: 1g
Sugar: 20g

Grandmother's Pie

Preparation time: 20 minutes Cooking time: 50-60 minutes Difficulty: Intermediate Servings: 8-10

Ingredients: For the crust:

- 2 cups all-purpose flour
- 1/2 teaspoon salt
- 1/2 cup unsalted butter, cold and cubed
- 4-5 tablespoons ice water

For the filling:

- 4 cups sliced apples (about 4-5 medium-sized apples)
- 1/2 cup granulated sugar
- 1/4 cup all-purpose flour
- 1 teaspoon ground cinnamon
- 1/4 teaspoon ground nutmeg
- 1/4 teaspoon salt
- 1 tablespoon lemon juice
- 2 tablespoons unsalted butter, melted

For the topping:

- 1/2 cup all-purpose flour
- 1/2 cup granulated sugar
- 1/4 cup unsalted butter, softened

Instructions:

1. Preheat the oven to 375°F (190°C).
2. In a large mixing bowl, whisk together the flour and salt for the crust. Add the cold cubed butter and use a pastry cutter or your fingers to cut it into the flour until the mixture resembles coarse crumbs.
3. Gradually add the ice water, one tablespoon at a time, and mix until the dough comes together. Be careful not to overmix. Form the dough into a ball, wrap it in plastic wrap, and refrigerate for 30 minutes.

4. Roll out the chilled dough on a lightly floured surface to fit a 9-inch pie dish. Transfer the rolled-out dough to the pie dish, pressing it gently into the bottom and sides. Trim any excess dough and crimp the edges.
5. In a large mixing bowl, combine the sliced apples, granulated sugar, flour, cinnamon, nutmeg, salt, and lemon juice for the filling. Toss until the apples are well coated.
6. Pour the apple filling into the prepared pie crust and drizzle the melted butter over the top.
7. In a separate bowl, combine the flour and sugar for the topping. Cut in the softened butter until the mixture resembles coarse crumbs.
8. Sprinkle the topping evenly over the apple filling.
9. Place the pie on a baking sheet to catch any drips and bake in the preheated oven for 50-60 minutes, or until the crust is golden brown and the filling is bubbly.
10. Remove the pie from the oven and let it cool on a wire rack for at least 1 hour before serving.
11. Slice and serve Grandmother's Pie on its own or with a scoop of vanilla ice cream or a dollop of whipped cream, and enjoy!

Nutritional values (per serving):

Calories: 320

Carbohydrates: 50g

Fat: 13g

Protein: 3g

Fiber: 3g

Sugar: 27g

Sweet Chocolate Pizza

Preparation time: 20 minutes Cooking time: 15-20 minutes Difficulty: Intermediate Servings: 8-10

Ingredients: For the pizza dough:

- 2 1/2 cups all-purpose flour
- 2 tablespoons granulated sugar
- 1 teaspoon instant yeast
- 1/2 teaspoon salt
- 1 cup warm water
- 2 tablespoons olive oil

For the chocolate sauce:

- 1 cup semisweet chocolate chips

- 1/2 cup heavy cream

For the toppings:

- 1 cup sliced strawberries
- 1/2 cup raspberries
- 1/4 cup chopped nuts (such as almonds or hazelnuts)
- Powdered sugar for dusting (optional)

Instructions:

1. Preheat the oven to 425°F (220°C).
2. In a mixing bowl, combine the flour, sugar, yeast, and salt for the pizza dough.
3. Gradually add the warm water and olive oil to the dry ingredients. Mix until a dough forms.
4. Transfer the dough to a floured surface and knead for about 5 minutes, or until the dough is smooth and elastic.
5. Place the dough in a greased bowl, cover it with a clean kitchen towel, and let it rise in a warm place for about 1 hour, or until doubled in size.
6. Meanwhile, prepare the chocolate sauce by heating the heavy cream in a small saucepan until it just begins to simmer. Remove from heat and pour the hot cream over the chocolate chips. Let it sit for a minute, then whisk until smooth and well combined. Set aside to cool slightly.
7. Once the dough has risen, punch it down and transfer it to a greased 12-inch pizza pan. Use your hands to press and stretch the dough evenly across the pan.
8. Spread the prepared chocolate sauce evenly over the pizza dough, leaving a small border around the edges.
9. Arrange the sliced strawberries and raspberries on top of the chocolate sauce. Sprinkle the chopped nuts over the fruit.
10. Place the pizza in the preheated oven and bake for 15-20 minutes, or until the crust is golden brown.
11. Remove the pizza from the oven and let it cool for a few minutes. Optional: Dust the top with powdered sugar for added sweetness and presentation.
12. Slice and serve the Sweet Chocolate Pizza while still warm and gooey, and enjoy!

Nutritional values (per serving):

Calories: 320

Carbohydrates: 43g

Fat: 14g
Protein: 6g

Fiber: 3g
Sugar: 15g

Apricot Tart

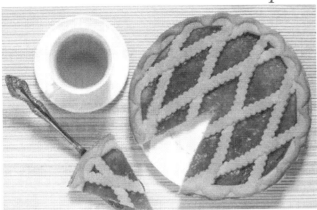

Preparation time: 30 minutes Cooking time: 40-45 minutes Difficulty: Intermediate Servings: 8-10

Ingredients: For the tart crust:

- 1 1/2 cups all-purpose flour
- 1/4 cup granulated sugar
- 1/4 teaspoon salt
- 1/2 cup unsalted butter, cold and cubed
- 1 egg yolk
- 2 tablespoons ice water

For the filling:

- 1 1/2 pounds fresh apricots, pitted and halved
- 1/4 cup apricot jam
- 2 tablespoons honey
- 1 tablespoon lemon juice
- 1 teaspoon vanilla extract

Instructions:

1. Preheat the oven to 375°F (190°C).
2. In a large mixing bowl, whisk together the flour, sugar, and salt for the tart crust. Add the cold cubed butter and use a pastry cutter or your fingers to cut it into the flour until the mixture resembles coarse crumbs.
3. In a small bowl, whisk together the egg yolk and ice water. Pour the egg mixture into the flour mixture and stir until the dough comes together. Form the dough into a ball, wrap it in plastic wrap, and refrigerate for 30 minutes.
4. Roll out the chilled dough on a lightly floured surface to fit a 9-inch tart pan. Transfer the rolled-out dough to the tart pan, pressing it gently into the bottom and up the sides. Trim any excess dough.
5. Arrange the apricot halves on top of the tart crust, cut side down.
6. In a small saucepan, heat the apricot jam, honey, lemon juice, and vanilla extract over medium heat until melted and well combined. Remove from heat.
7. Brush the apricot jam mixture over the apricot halves, ensuring they are evenly coated.
8. Place the tart in the preheated oven and bake for 40-45 minutes, or until the crust is golden brown and the apricots are tender.
9. Remove the tart from the oven and let it cool on a wire rack for at least 30 minutes before serving.
10. Serve the Apricot Tart at room temperature, either on its own or with a dollop of whipped cream or a scoop of vanilla ice cream, and enjoy!

Nutritional values (per serving):

Calories: 250
Carbohydrates: 38g
Fat: 10g

Protein: 3g
Fiber: 2g
Sugar: 20g

Lemon-Flavored Sweet Rice Fritters

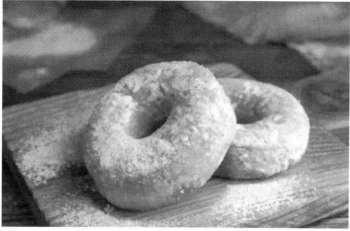

Preparation time: 20 minutes Cooking time: 20 minutes Difficulty: Intermediate Servings: 4

Ingredients:

- 1 cup cooked short-grain rice
- 1/4 cup all-purpose flour
- 2 tablespoons granulated sugar
- Zest of 1 lemon
- 1/2 teaspoon baking powder
- 1/4 teaspoon salt
- 1/4 cup unsweetened almond milk (or any non-dairy milk)
- 1 tablespoon lemon juice
- Vegetable oil, for frying
- Powdered sugar, for dusting

Instructions:

1. In a mixing bowl, combine the cooked rice, all-purpose flour, granulated sugar, lemon zest, baking powder, and salt.
2. Add the almond milk and lemon juice to the mixture. Stir well until all the ingredients are combined and you have a thick batter.
3. Heat vegetable oil in a deep frying pan or skillet over medium heat.
4. Using a spoon or ice cream scoop, drop small portions of the batter into the hot oil, making sure not to overcrowd the pan.
5. Fry the fritters for 2-3 minutes on each side, or until they turn golden brown and crispy.
6. Remove the fritters from the oil and place them on a paper towel-lined plate to absorb any excess oil.
7. Repeat the frying process with the remaining batter.
8. Once all the fritters are cooked and drained, transfer them to a serving platter.
9. Dust the fritters generously with powdered sugar.
10. Serve the Lemon-Flavored Sweet Rice Fritters warm as a delightful dessert or snack.

Nutritional values (per serving):

Calories: 180

Carbohydrates: 38g

Fat: 1g

Protein: 3g

Fiber: 1g

Sugar: 9g

Lemon Cheesecake

Preparation time: 20 minutes Chilling time: 4 hours or overnight Difficulty: Intermediate Servings: 8-10

Ingredients: For the crust:

- 1 1/2 cups graham cracker crumbs
- 1/4 cup granulated sugar
- 1/2 cup unsalted butter, melted

For the filling:

- 24 ounces (680g) cream cheese, softened
- 1 cup granulated sugar
- 3 large eggs
- 1/2 cup sour cream
- 1/4 cup fresh lemon juice
- Zest of 2 lemons
- 1 teaspoon vanilla extract

For the topping:

- 1 cup heavy cream
- 2 tablespoons powdered sugar
- Lemon zest, for garnish

Instructions:

1. Preheat the oven to 325°F (163°C).
2. In a medium bowl, combine the graham cracker crumbs, granulated sugar, and melted butter for the crust. Stir until the mixture resembles wet sand.
3. Press the crumb mixture into the bottom of a 9-inch springform pan, spreading it evenly. Press down firmly to create a compact crust.
4. In a large mixing bowl, beat the cream cheese and granulated sugar until smooth and creamy.
5. Add the eggs, one at a time, beating well after each addition.
6. Add the sour cream, lemon juice, lemon zest, and vanilla extract. Beat until all the ingredients are well incorporated and the mixture is smooth.
7. Pour the filling over the crust in the springform pan, spreading it evenly.
8. Bake in the preheated oven for 50-55 minutes, or until the center is set and the edges are slightly golden.
9. Remove the cheesecake from the oven and let it cool in the pan for 10 minutes. Then, run a knife around the edges of the pan to loosen the cheesecake.
10. Refrigerate the cheesecake for at least 4 hours or overnight to chill and set.
11. Just before serving, prepare the topping by whipping the heavy cream and powdered sugar together until stiff peaks form.
12. Remove the chilled cheesecake from the pan and transfer it to a serving plate.
13. Spread the whipped cream topping over the cheesecake.
14. Garnish with fresh lemon zest.
15. Slice and serve the Lemon Cheesecake chilled.

Nutritional values (per serving):

Calories: 480

Carbohydrates: 39g

Fat: 34g

Protein: 7g

Fiber: 1g

Sugar: 28g

28 DAY MEAL PLAN
Week 1

Day 1:
- Breakfast: Apples Pancakes
- Snack: Greek yogurt with fruit and granola
- Lunch: Zucchini Lasagna
- Snack: Peanut Butter Energy Bars
- Dinner: Chicken and Vegetable Penne with Walnut Parsley Pesto

Day 2:
- Breakfast: Porridge with banana and chocolate
- Snack: Veggie Sticks with Hummus
- Lunch: Quinoa Salad with Chicken and Avocado
- Snack: No-Bake Almond Date Bars
- Dinner: Chicken Stir-Fry with Brown Rice

Day 3:
- Breakfast: Walnut banana muffins
- Snack: Baked Kale Chips
- Lunch: Grilled Chicken and Vegetable Kabobs
- Snack: Savoury Basil Biscuits
- Dinner: Mushroom and Chicken Risotto

Day 4:
- Breakfast: Fruit and vegetable smoothie
- Snack: Sweet Beetroot Cake
- Lunch: Greek Salad with Grilled Shrimp
- Snack: Berry Protein Smoothie
- Dinner: Beef Stir-Fry with Broccoli and Brown Rice

Day 5:
- Breakfast: Whole wheat toast with peanut butter and banana
- Snack: Energy Balls
- Lunch: Turkey and Avocado Wrap
- Snack: Coconut Milk Rolls
- Dinner: Mexican-Style Lamb Tacos with Avocado Salsa

Day 6:
- Breakfast: Oatmeal and banana pancakes
- Snack: Veggie Sticks with Hummus
- Lunch: Lemon and Garlic Chicken Pasta
- Snack: Savory herb pancakes
- Dinner: Italian-Style Lamb Meatballs with Zucchini Noodles

Day 7:
- Breakfast: Chia seed pudding
- Snack: No-Bake Almond Date Bars
- Lunch: Grilled Chicken with Tomato and Cucumber Salad
- Snack: Lemon Blueberry Cake
- Dinner: Grilled Salmon with Mango Salsa

Week 2

Day 8:
- Breakfast: Carrot walnut muffins
- Snack: Baked Kale Chips
- Lunch: Stuffed Bell Peppers with Ground Turkey and Brown Rice

- Snack: Peanut Butter Energy Bars
- Dinner: Orange risotto with swordfish and shrimp

Day 9:
- Breakfast: Pineapple smoothie
- Snack: Veggie Sticks with Hummus
- Lunch: Chicken and Broccoli Alfredo Pasta
- Snack: Coconut Milk Rolls
- Dinner: Roasted Vegetables with Goat Cheese Polenta

Day 10:
- Breakfast: Cinnamon cake
- Snack: Energy Balls
- Lunch: Mediterranean Quinoa Chicken Bowl
- Snack: Savoury Basil Biscuits
- Dinner: Light Eggplant Parmesan

Day 11:
- Breakfast: French toast with fresh berries
- Snack: No-Bake Almond Date Bars
- Lunch: Whole Wheat Penne with Grilled Chicken and Roasted Vegetables
- Snack: Lemon Blueberry Cake
- Dinner: Mushroom and Chicken Risotto

Day 12:
- Breakfast: Carrot and Almond Cake
- Snack: Veggie Sticks with Hummus
- Lunch: Fish and Spinach Lasagna
- Snack: Berry Protein Smoothie
- Dinner: Chicken Stir-Fry with Brown Rice

Day 13:
- Breakfast: Golden Oatmeal Waffles with Blueberry Compote
- Snack: Baked Kale Chips
- Lunch: Roasted Vegetable and Quinoa Salad
- Snack: Coconut Milk Rolls
- Dinner: Stuffed Squid

Day 14:
- Breakfast: Lemon and Garlic Chicken Pasta
- Snack: Energy Balls
- Lunch: Greek Salad with Chicken
- Snack: Savory herb pancakes
- Dinner: Beetroot Savory Pie

Week 3

Day 15:
- Breakfast: Apple, Pear, and Cinnamon Smoothie
- Snack: Peanut Butter Energy Bars
- Lunch: Zucchini Lasagna
- Snack: Veggie Sticks with Hummus
- Dinner: Cauliflower Casserole

Day 16:
- Breakfast: Pumpkin Fritters
- Snack: No-Bake Almond Date Bars
- Lunch: Quinoa and Black Bean Stuffed Bell Peppers
- Snack: Coconut Milk Rolls
- Dinner: Fish and Spinach Lasagna

Day 17:
- Breakfast: Sweet Pumpkin Pancakes
- Snack: Baked Kale Chips
- Lunch: Chicken and Vegetable Penne with Walnut Parsley Pesto
- Snack: Savoury Basil Biscuits
- Dinner: White Zucchini Parmigiana

Day 18:
- Breakfast: Greek Yogurt with Fruit and Granola
- Snack: Energy Balls
- Lunch: Grilled Chicken with Tomato and Cucumber Salad
- Snack: Lemon Blueberry Cake
- Dinner: Cabbage Rolls with Baked Potatoes

Day 19:
- Breakfast: Whole Wheat Toast with Peanut Butter and Banana
- Snack: Veggie Sticks with Hummus
- Lunch: Lemon Garlic Shrimp Pasta
- Snack: Coconut Milk Rolls
- Dinner: Quinoa-Stuffed Bell Peppers

Day 20:
- Breakfast: Oatmeal and Banana Pancakes
- Snack: Baked Kale Chips
- Lunch: Mushroom and Chicken Risotto
- Snack: No-Bake Almond Date Bars
- Dinner: Beef Stir-Fry with Broccoli and Brown Rice

Day 21:
- Breakfast: Golden Oatmeal Waffles with Blueberry Compote
- Snack: Energy Balls
- Lunch: Roasted Vegetable and Quinoa Salad
- Snack: Savory Herb Pancakes
- Dinner: Mediterranean Quinoa Chicken Bowl

Week 4

Day 22:
- Breakfast: Berry Protein Smoothie
- Snack: Peanut Butter Energy Bars
- Lunch: Lemon Herb Chicken and Whole Wheat Orzo Salad
- Snack: Veggie Sticks with Hummus
- Dinner: Fish Couscous

Day 23:
- Breakfast: Apple, Pear, and Cinnamon Smoothie
- Snack: Baked Kale Chips
- Lunch: Greek Salad with Grilled Shrimp
- Snack: Coconut Milk Rolls
- Dinner: Pad Thai with Shrimp

Day 24:
- Breakfast: Pumpkin Fritters
- Snack: No-Bake Almond Date Bars
- Lunch: Warm Potato and Octopus Salad with Sweet Potatoes
- Snack: Savory Basil Biscuits
- Dinner: Stuffed Squid

Day 25:
- Breakfast: Greek Yogurt with Fruit and Granola

- Snack: Energy Balls
- Lunch: Grilled Salmon with Mango Salsa
- Snack: Lemon Blueberry Cake
- Dinner: Baked Salmon with Lemon and Herbs

Day 26:

- Breakfast: Whole Wheat Toast with Peanut Butter and Banana
- Snack: Baked Kale Chips
- Lunch: Chicken Stir-Fry with Brown Rice
- Snack: Coconut Milk Rolls
- Dinner: Roasted Vegetables with Goat Cheese Polenta

Day 27:

- Breakfast: Oatmeal and Banana Pancakes
- Snack: Energy Balls
- Lunch: Chickpea Burgers
- Snack: No-Bake Almond Date Bars
- Dinner: Light Eggplant Parmesan

Day 28:

- Breakfast: Golden Oatmeal Waffles with Blueberry Compote
- Snack: Veggie Sticks with Hummus
- Lunch: Quinoa and Black Bean Stuffed Bell Peppers
- Snack: Coconut Milk Rolls
- Dinner: Mediterranean Quinoa Chicken Bowl

CONCLUSION

In conclusion, the DASH Diet Cookbook is far more than just a collection of recipes; it is a comprehensive guide to adopting a healthier lifestyle that couldn't have come at a more opportune moment. Research unequivocally supports the effectiveness of DASH (Dietary Approaches to Stop Hypertension) principles in reducing blood pressure, promoting heart health, and enhancing overall well-being. So, why delay? It's time to set the culinary stage in your kitchen and treat your taste buds to a delightful array of flavor-packed dishes. Simultaneously, you're taking charge of your long-term health and well-being.

This cookbook offers a cornucopia of culinary delights, each masterfully crafted with both nutrition and taste in mind. From delectable breakfasts to vibrant salads, hearty soups, sensational main courses, and delightful desserts, the recipes within these pages prove that you need not compromise flavor for nutrition. The DASH Diet has never been so palate-pleasing!

The appeal of the DASH Diet extends beyond its mouthwatering recipes. It fosters a conscious and mindful approach to eating by reducing sodium, added sugars, and saturated fats while promoting portion control. This means you can relish a diverse array of foods while maintaining your weight. It's the dream come true!

This well-balanced diet benefits your body both inside and out. By embracing the DASH Diet, you are genuinely taking control of your long-term health and well-being. Rather than blindly following fleeting fads or restrictive eating plans, you're trading unhealthy fare for nourishing ingredients rich in essential nutrients that help your body function at its best. On the DASH Diet, there's no need for deprivation or rigid rules. It's about making sustainable and realistic lifestyle changes.

Discover the joy of experimenting with new flavors, relishing the natural tastes of unprocessed ingredients, and viewing food as a source of nourishment for both your body and soul. Food can indeed be a form of medicine! As you embark on this thrilling culinary adventure with the DASH Diet Cookbook, savor each bite and acknowledge the nourishment it provides. With every delectable meal, you are taking significant steps towards a healthier and happier lifestyle. Make this cookbook your trusted companion on the journey to improved health, where every scrumptious dish enhances your well-being. Here's to your vitality and cheerfully good health on your lifelong journey!

SHOPPING LIST

PRODUCE:
- Apples
- Bananas
- Basil leaves
- Blueberries
- Carrots
- Celery
- Cherry tomatoes
- Fennel
- Garlic
- Green beans
- Kale
- Lemon
- Mango
- Mushrooms
- Octopus
- Onion
- Orange
- Peppers (bell peppers and chili peppers)
- Potatoes
- Rocket (arugula)
- Spinach
- Squash (spaghetti squash and butternut squash)
- Sweet potatoes
- Tomatoes
- Zucchini

GRAINS AND BREADS:
- Whole wheat pasta
- Whole wheat bread
- Oatmeal
- Quinoa
- Rice (Venus rice)
- Lasagna noodles
- Linguine
- Spaghetti
- Couscous
- Polenta
- Flour (all-purpose and whole wheat)

PROTEIN:
- Chicken (breasts, thighs, ground chicken, sausage)
- Turkey (ground turkey, turkey breast)
- Lamb (ground lamb, lamb meatballs)
- Fish (tuna, swordfish, shrimp, cod, salmon, squid)
- Seitan
- Tofu
- Lentils
- Chickpeas
- Beans (black beans)
- Eggs

DAIRY AND ALTERNATIVES:
- Greek yogurt (vegan or regular)
- Nutritional yeast (vegan alternative to cheese)
- Almond milk
- Vegan cheese (optional)
- Vegan butter (optional)

NUTS AND SEEDS:
- Walnuts
- Almonds
- Chia seeds

PANTRY STAPLES:
- Olive oil
- Coconut milk
- Nut butter (peanut butter)
- Cinnamon
- Vanilla extract
- Cocoa powder
- Baking powder
- Baking soda
- Salt
- Pepper
- Herbs and spices (turmeric, oregano, basil, parsley, thyme, paprika, cayenne pepper)

CONDIMENTS AND SAUCES:
- Pesto sauce
- Tomato sauce
- Soy sauce
- Balsamic vinegar
- Mustard
- Honey or maple syrup (optional)
- Salsa (optional)

SNACKS AND EXTRAS:
- Energy bars
- Hummus
- Dates
- Cereal
- Popcorn

CONVERSION CHART

Measurement Type	Conversion
Length	
1 inch (in)	2.54 centimeters (cm)
1 inch (in)	25.4 millimeters (mm)
1 foot (ft)	0.3048 meters (m)
1 yard (yd)	0.9144 meters (m)
1 mile	1.60934 kilometers (km)
1 nautical mile	1.852 kilometers (km)
Area	
1 square inch (sq in)	6.4516 square centimeters (sq cm)
1 square foot (sq ft)	0.092903 square meters (sq m)
1 square yard (sq yd)	0.836127 square meters (sq m)
1 acre	4046.86 square meters (sq m)
1 square mile (sq mi)	2.58999 square kilometers (sq km)
1 hectare (ha)	10,000 square meters (sq m)
Volume	
1 teaspoon (tsp)	5 milliliters (ml)
1 tablespoon (tbsp)	15 milliliters (ml)
1 fluid ounce (fl oz)	29.5735 milliliters (ml)
1 cup	236.588 milliliters (ml)
1 pint (pt)	473.176 milliliters (ml)
1 quart (qt)	946.353 milliliters (ml)
1 gallon (gal)	3.78541 liters (l)
1 cubic inch (cu in)	16.3871 cubic centimeters (cu cm)
1 cubic foot (cu ft)	0.0283168 cubic meters (cu m)
1 cubic yard (cu yd)	0.764555 cubic meters (cu m)
1 milliliter (ml)	0.033814 fluid ounces (fl oz)
1 liter (l)	33.814 fluid ounces (fl oz)
1 liter (l)	1000 cubic centimeters (cu cm)
Weight/Mass	
1 ounce (oz)	28.3495 grams (g)
1 pound (lb)	0.453592 kilograms (kg)
1 ton (short ton)	907.185 kilograms (kg)
1 ton (long ton)	1016.05 kilograms (kg)
1 metric ton (t)	1000 kilograms (kg)
1 gram (g)	0.035274 ounces (oz)
1 kilogram (kg)	2.20462 pounds (lb)
1 kilogram (kg)	1000 grams (g)
Temperature	
To convert Celsius (°C) to Fahrenheit (°F):	$°F = (°C \times 9/5) + 32$
To convert Fahrenheit (°F) to Celsius (°C):	$°C = (°F - 32) \times 5/9$
Time	
1 minute (min)	60 seconds (sec)
1 hour (hr)	60 minutes (min)
1 day	24 hours (hr)
1 week	7 days

1 month (average)	30.44 days
1 year (average)	365.25 days
Speed	
1 mile per hour (mph)	1.60934 kilometers per hour (kph)
1 knot	1.852 kilometers per hour (kph)
1 kilometer per hour (kph)	0.621371 miles per hour (mph)
Pressure	
1 atmosphere (atm)	101,325 pascals (Pa)
1 atmosphere (atm)	760 millimeters of mercury (mmHg)
1 atmosphere (atm)	14.6959 pounds per square inch (psi)
1 bar	100,000 pascals (Pa)
1 bar	750.062 torr
1 bar	14.5038 pounds per square inch (psi)
Energy	
1 calorie (cal)	4.184 joules (J)
1 kilocalorie (kcal)	4.184 kilojoules (kJ)
1 British thermal unit (BTU)	1055.06 joules (J)
1 kilowatt-hour (kWh)	3,600,000 joules (J)

Made in United States
Orlando, FL
20 March 2025

59673112R00063